Medicinal Herbs
for Immune Defense

Medicinal Herbs
for Immune Defense

**104 TRUSTED RECIPES FOR FIGHTING
COLDS, FLUS, FEVERS & MORE**

JJ Pursell

Timber Press
Portland, Oregon

Published in 2021 by Timber Press, Inc.
The Haseltine Building
133 S.W. Second Avenue, Suite 450
Portland, Oregon 97204-3527
timberpress.com

Printed in China
Text and cover design by Vincent James

ISBN 978-1-64326-066-2
Catalog records for this book are available from
the Library of Congress and the British Library.

Contents

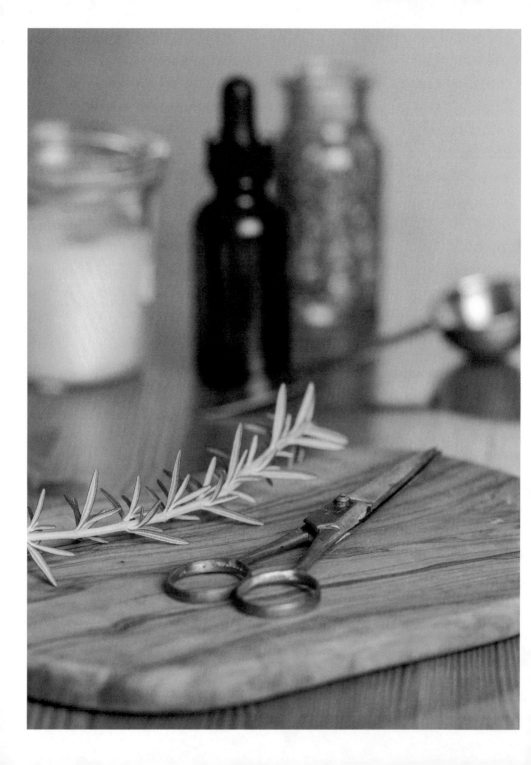

Introduction

Hello and welcome to an exploration of herbal medicine. This book, which is an abridged version of *Master Recipes for the Herbal Apothecary*, is intended as a resource for these troubling times. With the introduction of COVID-19 and the rise of novel viruses, we have found ourselves in unknown territory. Even those of us who research day in and day out have been left perplexed and often with more questions. Our immune systems, novel viruses, and the way the two interact create an ever-changing playing field, and it will most likely be years before we have a solid base of accurate information from which to make educated decisions.

In the meantime, we do what we know. Throughout the initial spread of COVID-19, I used herbs to keep myself and my family healthy. Sometimes my children would run from the room when certain tincture bottles from the regimen emerged, but I stuck to the foundations of my knowledge and we blessedly came out unscathed.

Protecting ourselves on the outside is the baseline of defense. The techniques of true hand washing, masks that minimize respiratory droplet exchange, gloves, changing of clothes, and social distancing all have solid research behind them. While nature cures and herbs have their limitations, using them to support our immune systems can provide a level of protection.

We exercise to keep our physical bodies strong and flexible. We choose healthy foods to optimize physical performance and vitalize our daily actions. And we take herbs as a preventative measure to support our organs and ensure they are functioning at their best. You can choose which herbs to take based on desired effects and intention, but you'll also want to ensure you are nourishing and considering the overall health of the individual.

This book is intended to provide general support to our innate immune systems. As research into new pathologies advances and new viruses are introduced into society, I encourage you to seek out accurate and reliable information. Some of my favorite resources are Kerry Bone, The Botanical Society of America, and Peter D'Adamo.

I have been reflecting on my experience over the last 20 years with patient and customer needs. Immune health is always a topic of conversation during fall and winter months. As cooler weather ushers people back inside and leads to the closing of windows, I gear up for the season's onslaught. Typically, I would know by December what "type" of year it was going to be. Some years were stomach flu years, others sinus colds or a rampant chest infection such as bronchitis. The trends were simple to follow and the information readily available. This allowed me to curate formulas and support my patients to the best of my ability.

In an age of antibiotic overuse and resistance, herbs offer our bodies support when faced with run-of-the-mill colds, flus, and foreign invasions. Antibiotics are best used to combat bacterial infections. Although they are ineffective in treating viruses, many people try to use them for this purpose anyway. In the past several decades, bacteria, viruses, and other organisms have advanced, figuring out new ways to overcome antibiotics and vaccines. If the host (your body) isn't providing the invader (a virus or bacteria) what it needs, the invader can mutate in an attempt to sneak around your defenses. More advanced invaders, such as the novel coronavirus, have learned to attack particular gateways on the cell to enable direct penetration of vital organs.

One of the best things we can do for these modern problems is to reacquaint ourselves with traditional herbal ways. Traditionally, yarrow is known to break fevers, boneset to ease the ache of flu, and sage to relieve a sore throat. Simple remedies of days long past offer an abundance of opportunities to care for ourselves and relieve suffering. Though I've been an herbalist for more than twenty-five years, I don't waiver in my daily practice of preventative care and am extremely diligent at the first sign of illness. I encourage you to adopt a daily practice that is feasible and protective.

As a motivated, creative go-getter type, I don't have the patience to be sick and, truth be told, I'm not a pleasant patient. I'm so sensitive that when even the slightest disturbance hits my body I need to go into shutdown mode. It's not something I can ignore or do my best to just get through. Instead, I attack whatever is attacking me, and I suggest you do the same.

A quick word about dehydration. When you're sick, sometimes it's hard enough just to lie in bed, let alone ensure you're drinking enough fluids. But upping your fluid intake is very important, especially if vomiting and/or diarrhea or thick congestion are present. Dehydration can sneak up on you, and before you know it, your decline is complicated by lack of hydration. When it sets in, you often feel extreme fatigue accompanied by any of the following: headache, dizziness, fever and chills, nausea, muscle cramps, or increased heart rate. Besides keeping you hydrated, upping your fluid intake breaks up excessive mucus, prevents constipation, reduces headaches, flushes the body of toxins, and keeps blood pressure normalized. If you've been vomiting and can't keep fluids down, taking sips of Replenish Herbal Tea every 15 minutes will help calm the stomach and open up the digestive process once again. And when I say sips, that's exactly what I mean. One tiny sip and then wait for a full 15 minutes. Any more than that can trigger the stomach to convulse and repel the healing fluids, especially if you've been in a vomiting spell.

One powerful reason for turning to herbal medicine is that it provides access to healing medicine on the spot, hours or days before you could even get a doctor's appointment. It gives the body a chance to hold steady through or potentially overcome an illness before we are able to access help from our practitioner.

How and why herbs work is something of an esoteric conversation. I could provide endless citations of scientific papers on the effects of specific plant constituents, but the total healing effect of an herb on the body is more than the sum of its parts. Let's take echinacea as an example. Echinacea is one of the most researched herbs, with most researchers isolating individual components of the root to identify what actions it produces in the body. This is the most common way for researchers to study an herb, by taking it apart and looking at each part (constituent) individually. The most prominent constituents of *Echinacea purpurea* are caffeic acid derivatives (phenolic compounds), alkamides, and polysaccharides. Research shows that caffeic acid derivatives are potent antioxidants that have important anti-inflammatory effects. Alkamides have stimulatory effects on phagocytosis (they destroy foreign cell types) and trigger effects on the pro-inflammatory cytokines. Cytokines are cell-signaling molecules that aid cell-to-cell communication in immune responses and stimulate the movement of cells toward sites of inflammation, infection, and trauma.

My point here is that research is a great way to identify the individual components of an herb and their actions. This serves an educational purpose and adds to the body of scientific knowledge about plants looked to by those who prefer to rely on science as they consider how to incorporate herbs into their lives. But, and I'm guessing you were feeling the *but* coming, the scientific research method misses a key point: herbs and the greater plant kingdom in general don't work because or when their specific components are isolated. Each plant has evolved a series of complex systems that work symbiotically when all parts function together.

It's possible, for example, for one herb to contain elements that individually have contradictory actions such as moistening and drying or astringing and dilating. It seems odd, perhaps, until you think that herbs must be self-sufficient to survive in the wild. They must have many different mechanisms in order to handle various conditions, and they turn to different parts of their own innate nature as needed to respond to them. Therein lies the magic and wisdom of nature.

One of the most frequent questions I hear from people beginning an herbal medicine regimen is: How does an herb know where it's needed in the body? Using our echinacea example again, someone might ask: How does it know to go to my nose and head to relieve cold symptoms? Well, an herb responds in much the same way as a pain reliever like Tylenol. Both are responding to messages the brain receives from the body. When you experience pain or symptoms in your body, certain chemicals are released. These chemicals contain messages and these messages are sent to the brain to alert it of what and where the issue is. When you take medicine, its goal is to find where the messages are coming from so it can help. Once it does, it turns off the chemical response, calms the reaction, and returns the physiological function back to normal. It also offers healing constituents to do its best to correct the problem. This is where the multitude of varying actions really shine. Whereas a drug often has one action, an herb can offer many different supporting actions. And if you blend herbs together—for example, echinacea and myrrh, traditionally used to treat pain and inflammation—you begin to create a dynamic medicinal force that can directly soothe your symptoms.

So what balance do you personally want to strike between letting science and experience guide your personal herbal journey? Perhaps you want to get deep into herbs' biological constituents, learning classifications and their actions, in which case I'd refer you to my volume, *The Herbal Apothecary*. Or maybe you'd rather learn experientially, taking in a recommended plant as a tea or tincture and recording your personal experience with it. The more you use herbs, the more they will become like trusted friends you can call upon whenever you need them. Personally, I have a biochemistry past and have spent many years looking into plants' scientific natures, so thinking about the positive chemical interactions they can create reinforces what folk and ethnic practitioners have long dictated. As with any passion that lasts a lifetime, the body of knowledge you'll accumulate through your own practice will become a part of you and your daily life.

Master Recipes

The first step in learning how to use herbs effectively as medicine is educating yourself about the various ways they can be applied or ingested. This chapter details the most common ways to use herbs. Different preparations are recommended for different conditions. If I need headache relief quickly, I choose a tincture, because it enters the bloodstream quickly, whereas if my stomach is upset I typically drink a cup of soothing tea. First I'll discuss various types of herbal products—teas, tinctures, oils, salves, and so forth. This will give you an idea of what each type is and whether it has an internal or external application. Then I'll go into detail about the process of making each one. I'll provide basic recipes so you can try your hand at making each product. Don't worry; it's much easier than you think! This section is important as it gives you pearls of information to be successful at making the recipes in the remainder of the book. With a little practice, you'll then be ready to make any recipe listed. After a while you may even decide to adapt the recipes to your preference and need.

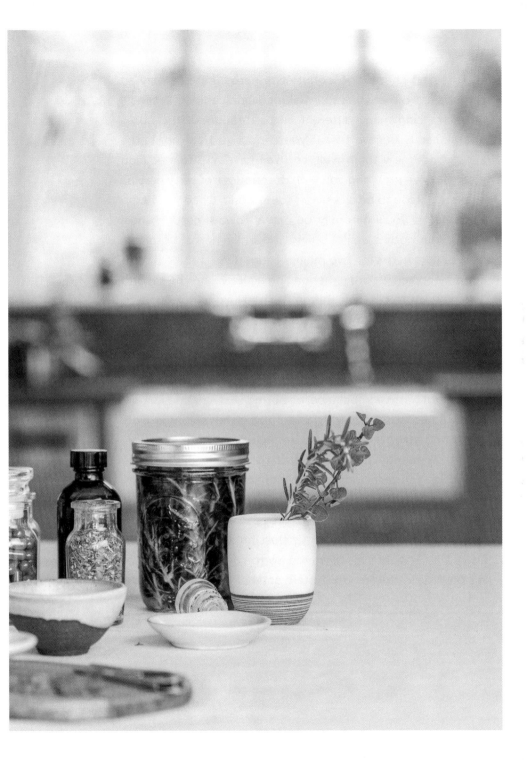

The next chapter describes sixty herbs that can play an essential part in anyone's herbal medicine cabinet. While I'll be referencing many different herbs throughout the book, I passionately believe that if you choose just twenty herbs and get to know them well, you will have all the medicine you need. I've provided you with descriptions of sixty here as some will prove to be allies, and some won't. Once you begin using herbs, you'll naturally be drawn toward certain ones. This is your body's way of telling you which herbs it prefers.

We take herbs for two main reasons. One is to help remedy a symptom we are experiencing acutely, and the second is to attempt to create a shift in the body from imbalance to balance. I will refer to these two types throughout the book as acute or chronic conditions. An acute condition refers to things like a sprained ankle or simple headache. Examples of chronic conditions are inflammation from an old injury, longstanding digestive imbalance, or hormone dysregulation.

One question frequently asked about the recipes is: How much do I take? If you are experiencing an acute situation, dosing frequently is more important than dosing in large quantities. Frequent dosing of small amounts sends a powerful message of consistency to the problem at hand that it needs to change. Dosing 1 or 2 dropperfuls of tincture or 1 cup of tea *every 2 to 3 hours* is best for acute dosing. Yes, every 2 to 3 hours. This gives the body a consistent bump of support to strengthen the system and help it regain balance.

For a chronic condition, take a small dose for a period of time, 4 to 12 weeks depending on the condition, to work with the body to create a sustained physical change. Typically the dose is 1 dropperful of tincture 2 to 3 times per day, or 2 to 3 cups of tea a day. Common dosing times are morning and night or morning, midday, and night. Think of it this way. If you've experienced chronic constipation for years, how long do you think it will take to heal the cause of what started that problem? One day? One week? Most likely not. Give it time. Herbs generally work to restore function and integrity of the body, which is not a quick fix. Give the herbs time to help the body return to a state of balance and the tissues the chance to return to a state of integrity and proper function. We ask a lot of our bodies. By giving your body this consistent attention, you can return it to health.

Types of Preparations, Uses & Basic Dosages for Adults

PREPARATION	TARGETS	CHRONIC OR TONIC DOSAGE	ACUTE DOSAGE
capsule	various conditions	2 capsules 1 or 2 times a day	2 or 3 capsules 3 or 4 times a day
essential oil blend	various conditions	typically used for acute conditions	1 to 5 drops as needed
flower essence blend	emotional and psychological health	4 drops 4 times a day	4 drops 4 times a day
fomentation	sprains, strains, pain, broken bones	typically used for acute conditions	enough to saturate a cloth slightly larger than affected area, applied 1 to 3 times a day for 20 minutes
herbal oil	skin conditions, pain, colic, lymph congestion, soreness, overall anxiety	enough to cover affected area, applied 1 to 3 times a day	enough to cover affected area, applied 1 to 3 times a day
medicinal tea	all physical conditions	2 to 3 cups a day for 4 to 12 weeks	1 cup every 2 to 3 hours as needed

PREPARATION	TARGETS	CHRONIC OR TONIC DOSAGE	ACUTE DOSAGE
poultice	stings, wounds, broken bones, sprains, skin conditions	typically used for acute conditions	enough to cover affected area, applied 1 or 2 times a day
salve	burns, cuts, scrapes, stress, pain	typically used for acute conditions	enough to cover affected area, applied repeatedly until pain ceases
spray	blue moods, emotional conditions, inflammation, cuts, sore throat	typically used for acute conditions	spritz as needed or 1 to 2 sprays for physical conditions
syrup	colds and coughs, headaches, upset stomach, hair and scalp conditions	typically used for acute conditions	1 to 2 teaspoons 1 to 3 times a day
tincture	all physical conditions	1 dropperful 2 to 3 times a day for 4 to 12 weeks	1 to 2 dropperfuls every 2 to 3 hours as needed
wash	skin conditions, eye infections, wounds, post partum	typically used for acute conditions	1 quart used 1 or 2 times a day

A note about quantities: All the tea recipes will result in 4 ounces of loose tea. This is a standard amount and enough to make blending slightly easier. If you want to make a smaller amount, feel free to halve or quarter the recipe to begin. Tincture recipes will be created in quantities of 1 or 2 ounces, with 1 ounce of tincture equaling 30 milliliters of fluid, and 2 ounces, 60 milliliters. Capsule recipes will result in 200 capsules, and again you can reduce or double any recipe to fit your needs. All of the herbs called for in this book are to be used in dried form unless noted otherwise.

The best advice I can give is to dive right in. Read through all the material then give it a go. Try mixing a tea or applying a poultice for practice. The quickest way to learn is through experimentation, and the best way to learn about the herbs is to use them and to take note of how the remedies help you achieve acute symptom relief or a better balance of daily health.

I encourage you to try the recipes that seem appealing or relate to a condition or issue you've struggled with. You can read about herbs all day long, but until you actually use them, you truly haven't learned anything! Just like learning anything new, using herbs for the first time can feel scary or bring up feelings of uncertainty, both of which are completely normal. The first time I tried to blend a tea, it was so bitter I had to laugh and throw it out. Expect to experience a trial-and-error period until you have a foundation underneath you.

A final note: this book is focused on recipes for those who want to make their own medicine. If you'd rather not do it yourself but want the end result of one of the recipes listed, you can always call your local herb shop to have them blend the recipe for you.

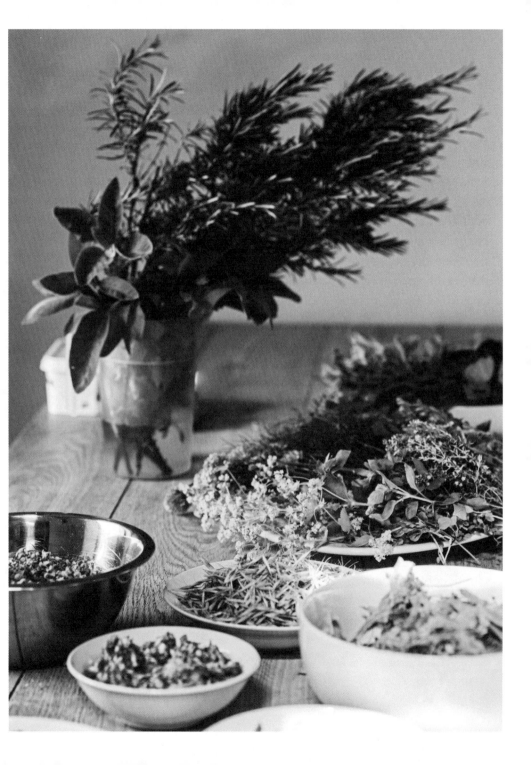

Key Kitchen Supplies

Here are some things you'll want to have on hand for preparing the recipes. Before you begin, sterilize all your cookware and storage containers to reduce the risk of bacterial and fungal contamination. Use the sterile mode in your dishwasher or place the items in boiling water. All your storage containers should be thoroughly dry before use. This little tip will help to ensure that your medicine lasts longer and stays fresher.

- aluminum foil
- baking dish
- calculator
- cheesecloth
- coffee filters
- coffee or nut grinder
- cooking brush or paint-brush
- cooking thermometer
- crockpot
- fine-mesh strainers, small, medium, and large
- funnels, small, medium, and large
- glass containers, quart-size with secure lids
- mason jars, pint- and quart-size
- measuring cups, small, medium, and large
- mixing bowls
- mixing spoons
- muddling bar
- notebook
- packing rod
- pencil
- percolation vessel
- plastic sandwich bags
- rocks or paperweights
- rubber bands
- saucepan, stainless steel or ceramic
- shot glass
- soaking basin
- stockpot, stainless steel or ceramic
- Vitamix blender
- waxed paper

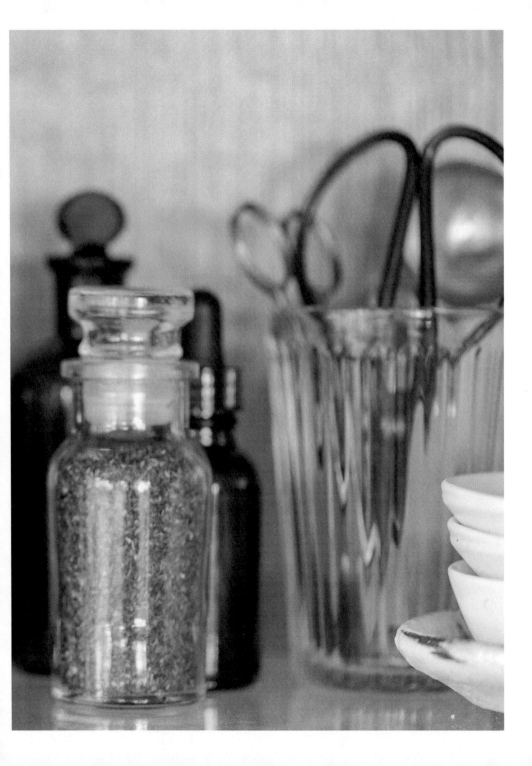

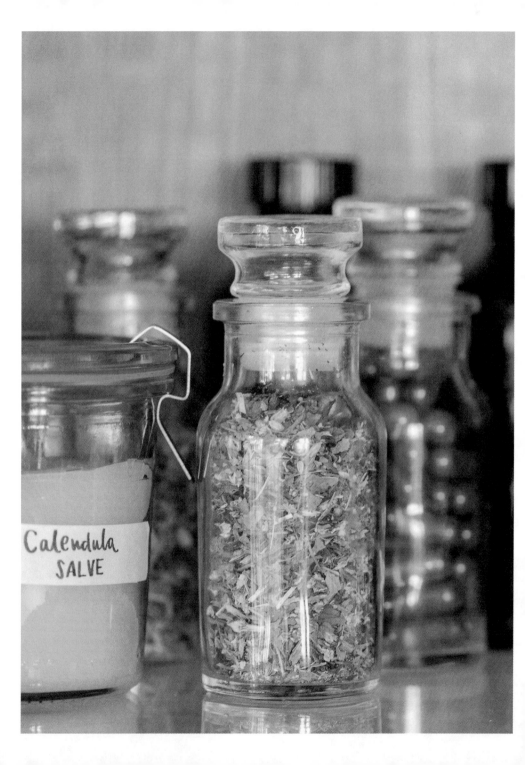

Capsules

I've been amazed throughout my years as an herbalist by my customers' love of taking pills. Capsules are easy, convenient, and travel well. They also have no taste, which seems to be a big plus for many people. I also think because the supplement market is now mainstream that taking capsules and tablets is widely accepted as normal, and they are easier for many people to keep around than herbal tinctures and salves. While capsules and tablets are accessible and easy to transport, they are not always the best option. Anyone who is experiencing digestive imbalance, for example, might not be able to reap capsules' full benefit if they already have an inability to break food down properly. This can be due to a lack of digestive enzymes, digestive tract inflammation, or perhaps the material used to contain the capsule or bind the tablet. I encourage my patients to consider other modes of medicine transmission when the digestive system is challenged. There is nothing worse than wasting money on something you are hoping will work but that your body isn't able to utilize.

One thing is for sure, though—herbal capsules are extremely easy to make. You really do want to use herbal powder, as this will make the whole process much easier and quicker. You can grind the dried herb, but unless you've got an amazing herb grinder that can really get it to a powder level, I suggest purchasing prepared herb powder. Then you need to choose between two capsule materials: gelatin and

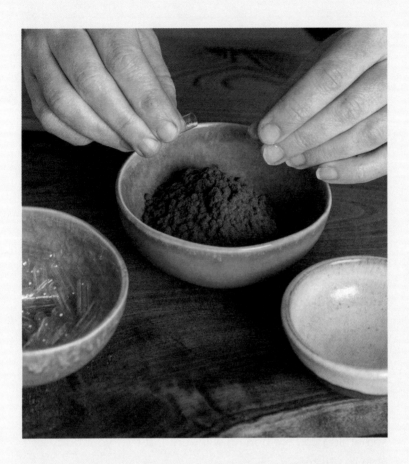

vegetable glycerin. Gelatin is cheaper, but I prefer the natural substance of vegetable glycerin. The other thing to be aware of is that empty capsules come in varying sizes: 0 (the smallest), 00, and 000 (the largest). To help you visualize, my daughter calls 000 capsules "horse pills."

If you want to create a blend of different herbs for yourself, write out your blend and determine the proportions of each herb. Weigh them out and mix together before encapsulating.

Basic Capsule Recipe

2 ounces powdered herb(s)

200 empty capsules

Place the powdered herbs in the capsules using either the homestyle method or a capsule maker. For homestyle, follow these steps:

1. Put the herbal powder in a bowl. Approximately 2 ounces will make 200 capsules, give or take depending on the capsule size.

2. Separate a capsule and scoop herbal powder from the bowl into each side of the capsule. It's like a diving-for-herb-powder experience. Your fingers will get a little dirty.

3. Close the capsule. Careful not to overfill or you won't be able to close it.

If you'd rather invest in a capsule maker, such as a Cap-M-Quik, they are very easy to use and you can make 200 capsules very quickly. Put the bottom part (the larger piece) of the capsule into the tray and then pour the powder onto the tray. Use the spreading tool to disperse the powder evenly and then gently tap it down. Once the capsules are filled, shake off the extra powder and lower the tray. The bottom parts of the capsules are exposed and all you need to do is stick on the tops.

At my herb shop, Fettle Botanic Supply & Counsel, I packaged my capsule products in paper canisters to keep the costs down so customers were only paying for the medicine. But, at home, I recommend you store your capsules in a glass jar and keep it away from heat and sunlight. This helps the capsules stay fresh for a long time.

Essential Oil Blends

Essential oils, which can be blended together or added to an herbal formula, are another way in which plants can offer healing. Essential oils are derived through extraction by one of the following methods: steam distillation, water distillation, solvent extraction, enfleurage, cold press extraction, or CO_2 extraction. These methods basically pull out the oils of the plant, and most yield both water and essential oil. The essential oil sits on top of the water, which after processing is called a hydrosol. The oil contains specific medicinal constituents, and the hydrosol (which smells lovely but has a lighter scent than the oil) has medicinal properties as well, but these are typically limited to the water-soluble aspects of the plant's constituents.

Some of the recipes in this book direct you to add essential oils to other ingredients for salves or herbal oils, and other recipes tell how to create essential oil blends targeting specific conditions. For blends consisting only of essential oils, essential oil quantities are indicated in milliliters since the typical essential oil bottle is 5 or 10 milliliters. If the essential oil blend involves using a carrier oil, the measurements are in drops of essential oil and ounces of carrier oil. Always use pure therapeutic essential oils in your healing recipes and be sure to keep the caps on the bottles. A pure essential oil will evaporate if the cap is left off. Read the ingredients to make sure your oils are not adulterated with carrier oils, fragrance, or perfume. The few exceptions would be the exotic essential

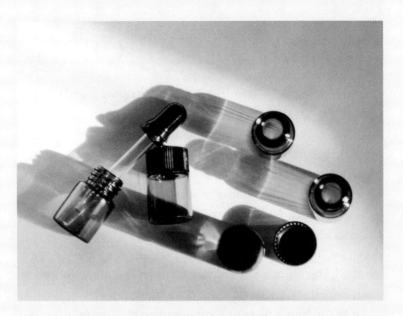

oils such as rose, neroli, and jasmine. These are often purchased in 5- or 10-percent dilutions to make them affordable.

Essential oils can be used in many ways, but I typically
don't recommend applying them directly to the skin, as they
can be quite caustic. If you want to use an essential oil topically, first dilute it with olive, apricot, or coconut oil. Some
essential oils, such as oregano, should never be used in direct
contact with the skin. They are best added to a vaporizer or
essential oil diffuser so that you are breathing in very small
amounts. Some essential oils are also beneficial in a bath or as
one or two drops on your pillow. And please keep in mind that
essential oils are very toxic to most animals, especially cats.

Fomentations

A fomentation is a strong herbal brew, similar to a wash, applied by soaking a cotton cloth in it and then placing the cloth on or wrapping it around the affected area. Heat is often added to help drive the herbs into the skin. Fomentations are perfect for applying to body parts that move or are not conducive to sitz baths or washes.

One of my favorite uses for fomentations is with my patients after any type of body treatment, whether it be acupuncture, massage, or an adjustment. Ending the appointment by placing a warm fomentation on the area worked on really sets the patient up for a good day. In a clinic I used to work at, we had a fomentation warming throughout the day so it was ready to use. The combination of herbs gave the clinic an aroma that evoked healing, and the patients loved the fomentation as it created a sense of calm, relaxation, and closure at the end of the visit.

For strains and sprains, a fomentation is an excellent first-line treatment. Areas like knees and elbows are perfect candidates for fomentations, as they are difficult to soak. Making a lavender and black cohosh fomentation for the nape of the neck can do wonders for headaches and stress. The next time loved ones are showing strain on their face or with their body language, surprise them with a fomentation treat.

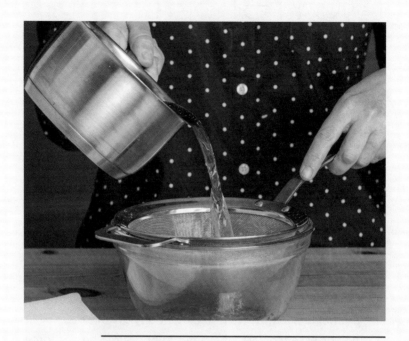

Basic Fomentation Recipe

6 tablespoons fresh or dried herbs

1 quart water

Mix the herbs with the water and steep one or two hours. Straint the herbs out and gently warm up in a saucepan on the stove on low. Soak a cotton cloth in the pan, wring it out, and apply to affected area.

Flower Essence Blends

While herbal medicine focuses primarily on the physical health of the human body, flower essences work subtly to balance our emotional layers. Repeatedly experiencing emotions such as fear, anger, or grief can divert us from making healthy choices and can also negatively affect us on a physical level. Working with our emotions with the help of flower essences can lead to overall health on multiple levels. We can put together a custom blend to help us with the emotional and mental challenges we're facing at any given time.

Flower essences are energetic imprints of the life force of plants that interact with our spiritual essences, helping to evoke specific qualities within us. Specific flower essences have affinities for particular emotions or blockage patterns, discovered through research and study. The Flower Essence Society (flowersociety.org) in California has been conducting research since 1979 and is the leading authority. The organization offers endless resources as well as classes and certifications, should you wish to learn more.

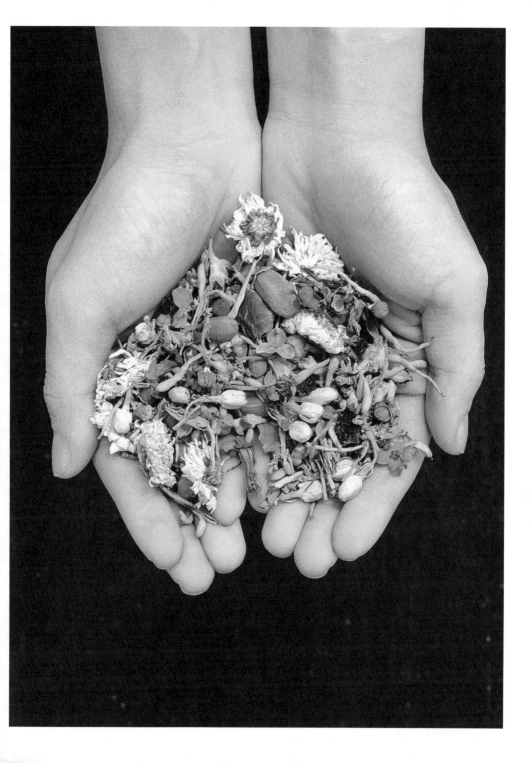

Herbal Oils

Many people I speak with confuse herbal oils with essential oils. To be clear, an herbal oil for our purposes is an herb-infused oil, most often olive oil, that can be used topically in that form or as the base of another herbal product such as a salve, a lotion, or a cream. An essential oil is a distilled product. Both are wonderful, but they are very different from one another. Herbal oils are yet another way to use herbs topically.

You may be asking yourself at this point: When would I use an oil versus a salve or a wash? Knowing what you are treating is the first step and so is understanding the qualities of the different herbal applications. Oils and salves are both wonderful for softening, soothing, and healing skin. They are great at pulling tissues together and treating the superficial layers as well as acting as a medium to carry things slightly deeper into the body. Oil is naturally absorbed through the skin, so if it has been infused with healing herbs, the oil-soluble constituents of the herb are absorbed as well. Oils are more readily absorbed into the body than lotions. Lotions often have additional ingredients that help them sit atop the skin, whereas oils drive into deeper skin levels. But an oil-based application is not always indicated. One example is with poison ivy or oak. With a poison ivy or oak outbreak on the skin, the oil in the plant is what causes the discomfort. Using an oil-based application will only provoke and spread the condition. When you need to cool down, flush, or soak the skin, a wash is indicated. As another example, using healing oils

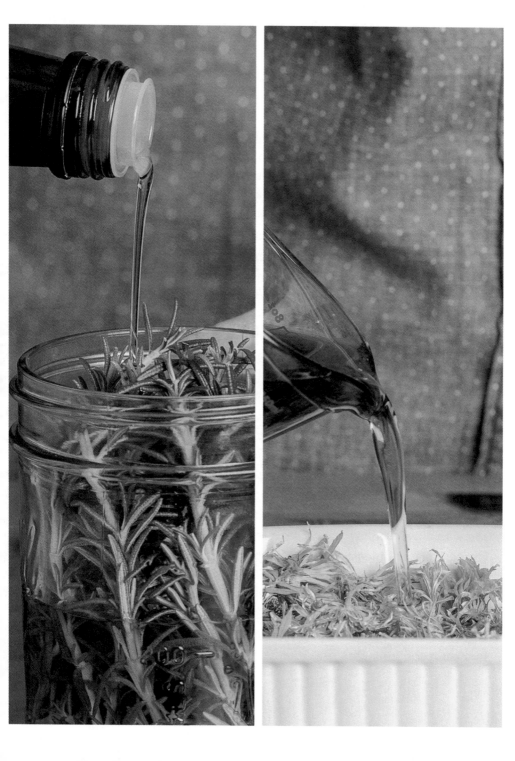

on the perineum may be helpful, but it prefers the cooling action of a water-based application.

Herbal oils are the base of many other herbal products including salves, lotions, creams, and lip balms. Making and having a couple of herbal oils on hand allows you the freedom to whip up something when you need it or when you are looking for a fun activity on a rainy day. I prefer to make oils with fresh plant material, but dried herbs can also be used in most cases. Making oils with fresh plants generates a yearlong ongoing cycle of herbal oil production based on the plants coming up or in bloom. As I'm writing this, the mullein flowers are making their appearance and I've just made a fresh batch of mullein flower oil. Seeing the bright yellow flowers submerged in olive oil as sunshine passes through the jar on my windowsill is something that brings me peace and joy each day.

While you can make most herbal oils with fresh or dried material, some can only be processed fresh: arnica flowers, mullein flowers, and St. John's wort flowers. When using fresh material I favor the folk method, or the herbalist way as I prefer to call it. Get a jar and fill it three quarters of the way full with your plant material. Don't pack the herb too tightly or the oil can't get through and around it all. Fill the jar to the top with olive oil, close it, and set it in the sun. A consistent temperature of at least 75 to 80 degrees F is best. Shake it daily and keep an eye out for water precipitate. If it looks murky on the bottom, that usually is water precipitate and you can use a turkey baster to draw it out as needed. You can also dump the entire contents into a saucepan and gently heat it for 5 minutes, and then put it back in the jar and continue sun steeping. Two weeks is the standard amount of time for sun steeping.

If you don't have consistent sun or are using dried herbs, the oven method will work. Place your herbs in a glass baking pan and add enough oil to cover the herbs 1 or 2 inches deep. Turn your oven on low, 170 to 200 degrees F, and bake the mixture for 4 to 6 hours. Keep an eye on it and ensure your oven isn't too hot. Stirring it from time to time is good too. Herbal oils made this way often end up with the herbs crispy and burnt looking. This is normal, as long as your oven wasn't too hot and your oil is not burnt. Strain into a glass jar and store the oil in a dark, cool place.

Basic Herbal Oil Recipe

fresh or dried herbs

olive oil

For fresh herbs, loosely fill a pint jar three quarters full of the herb and fill it to the top with olive oil. Close the lid and sun steep for 2 weeks.

For dried herbs, put the desired amount of the herb in a small glass baking pan and cover with olive oil to a depth of 1 or 2 inches. Bake at 170 to 200 degrees F in the oven, stirring occasionally, for 4 to 6 hours. Strain into a glass jar and store in a dark, cool place.

Liniments

Liniments are topical applications that can increase blood circulation and promote healing. Liniments are applied on unbroken skin and often used for sore muscles, aches, and pains. They differ from fomentations in that the solution is made with a solvent like isopropyl alcohol, witch hazel, or vinegar. Liniments penetrate and evaporate quickly on the skin's surface, but their actions can have lasting effects. A few liniment recipes are given in the book but are varied enough that I won't give a basic recipe here.

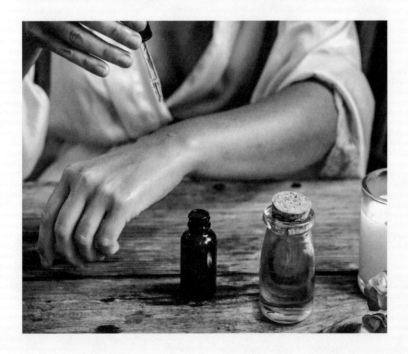

Medicinal Teas

Herbal teas, so often associated with specific flavors rather than specific medicinal effects, are unsung herbal heroes, able to create significant physiological changes in the body. It's hard not to say that every herb tea has medicinal value, in fact. Something considered as benign as chamomile tea can have significant effects on the body. I've seen women who regularly drink chamomile tea experience decreased menstrual cramping and more regulated cycles. Some people have a ritual of drinking peppermint tea after dinner simply because they like the taste and realize it cleanses the palate; they may not know that it became an after-dinner tradition because of the digestive support it offers.

Medicinal teas made from herbal blends can be brewed by the cup as needed or in batches designed to provide one day's worth of medicine. I don't recommend making herbal tea in larger batches, as many of the herbs don't keep well after a day or two. Even in the refrigerator, some herbs like slippery elm bark or marshmallow root will sour the tea once it is made or impart a bitter flavor. A batch is 1 quart or roughly 3 10-ounce cups of tea. You can make a quart of tea one of two ways. Both are equally fine; it's just a matter of preference and whether you need something immediately or can prepare ahead of time.

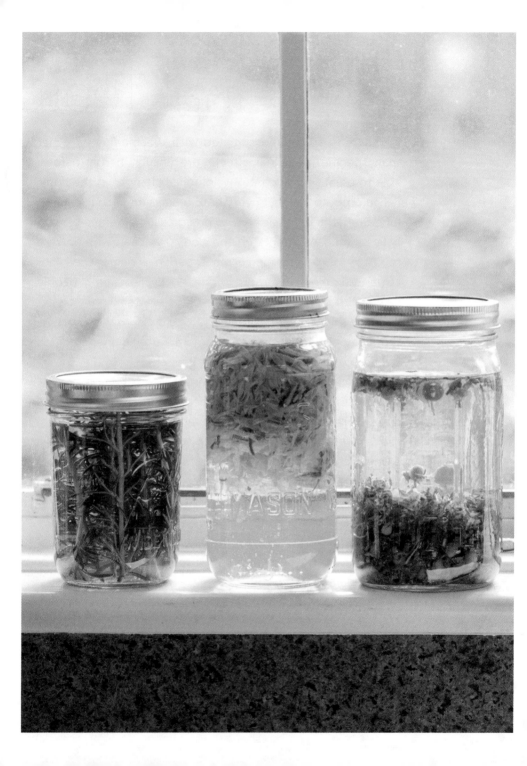

Medicinal Tea:
Quart Jar Method

Place 4 to 5 tablespoons of dried herbs in a quart jar. Set a full kettle of water on the stove and turn on the heat. Right before the water boils, or at around 200 degrees F, pull the kettle off the heat. After a while your ear will be trained to hear the almost boiling point. Pour the hot water over the herbs to almost the top of the jar. Close with the lid or place a tea towel over the top and let sit 4 hours or overnight. The hot water, combined with the longer steeping time, will work to steep all plant material types, whether leaves, roots, or flowers. Once steeping is complete, strain the tea. Divide this up into 3 cups for the day, drinking it hot or cold, depending on your mood, constitution, and personal preference.

Most often teas are steeped and drunk hot, but if a cooling effect is desired you can try drinking it cold. If you are dealing with a complaint like a phlegmy head cold, drinking it hot will aid the herbs' efforts. While most research shows drinking tea hot is more beneficial, an herb like marshmallow root is great cold to soothe bladder inflammation. And some teas such as marshmallow, slippery elm, chamomile, and blessed thistle are best steeped using cold water. These herbs have mucilage and/or bitter compounds that should be preserved and that to a small extent might be decreased with boiling water. Remember, cold-brewed tea is a natural diuretic, which means it can increase urination.

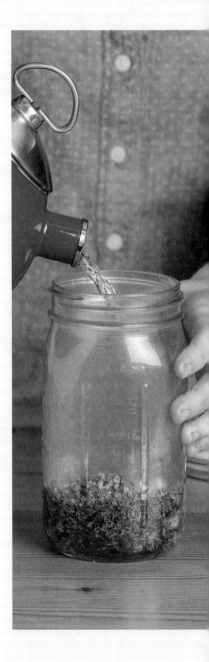

Medicinal Tea:
Stove Top Method

Sometimes you need a cup of medicinal tea quickly. In this case or if you prefer, you can make your medicinal tea on the stove top. With the quart jar method, it doesn't matter if you have leaves, flowers, roots, or bark, as the long duration of steeping allows all the constituents to be extracted. In the stove top method, the herb part determines the process. If you have an herbal blend that has roots and bark only, this process is quite easy. Simply put 1 quart plus 1/2 cup extra of water in a pot on your stove and turn on the heat. Once it begins to boil, turn it down to a simmer, add 4 to 5 tablespoons of herbs, and cover for 15 minutes. Ensure it is a light simmer. If the water is boiling, you'll lose too much of it in the process. After 15 minutes, turn off the heat and let cool slightly. Strain the tea.

If your tea consists of a combination of roots and flowers and leaves, you will need to complete an extra step. The more delicate parts of herbs such as flowers and leaves cannot tolerate high simmering heat, as it destroys their potency. Therefore, you'll complete the steps described in the previous paragraph, but once you turn off the heat, you'll add 1 more tablespoon of the herbal blend, give a quick stir, cover the pot back up, and let it steep for 10 to 15 minutes. This allows for infusion of the leaves and/or flowers into the water. Then you can strain the herbs from the water and enjoy.

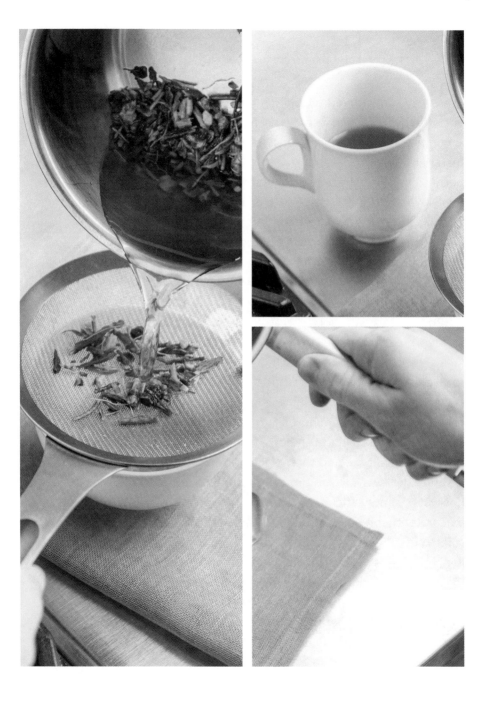

Poultices

I've always considered a poultice one of the most primitive yet effective ways to use herbs for healing. By definition, a poultice is a soft, damp mass of material, typically plant material or plant material mixed with flour, applied to the body to relieve soreness and inflammation. It's applied in a thick layer and kept in place with a cloth. You may have seen recommendations to add heat, but I haven't found that to be necessary in order for the poultice to be effective. Many times the natural heat of the body is sufficient.

You might have had a grandmother who sautéed onions and ginger whenever you had a cold. Not to eat, mind you, but to then mix with flour and stuff into an old sock to apply to your throat and neck. When I was a kid this was torture, but I really cannot think of a time when it didn't eventually put me to sleep and greatly reduce whatever cold was ailing me.

In both Western and Chinese herbalism, making an herb cake from fresh or dried herbs and applying it directly to the skin is common. Taking the herb, mixing it with a bit of hot water to open it up, and then placing it on the affected area is the easiest way. If you are out and about and don't have hot water, simply sticking the fresh herb into your mouth to macerate it works great too. Just ensure it's an herb that is safe to eat. The saliva actually does a good job of keeping it all together so it can then be spit out and held in place on the skin. I live on a farm, and we are outside a lot and fre-quently get splinters. Most of the time they are easy enough to pull out, but sometimes a poultice is needed to soften the surrounding skin so I can get ahold of the splinter. Using drawing herbs such as plantain and comfrey leaf can turn tears into smiles with my kids as we pick the leaves and chew to our hearts' content before spitting on each other. Letting the poultice sit for as little as five minutes usually draws out the tip of the splinter just enough to grasp it.

Practice making poultices in the following way so you are confident in their use when you need them. With dried or fresh herbs, mash just enough in a small bowl with a splash of hot water to cover the affected area. If using fresh, cut or tear into small pieces before mashing. Mash until the mixture has a pastelike consistency. Once it has cooled a bit, apply to the affected area. If you can relax for 15 to 20 minutes, do so and hold still so the poultice stays in place. If you need to be on the go, wrap with sterile gauze or cover with a large Band-Aid. You can leave the poultice on as long as it seems helpful, but keeping it clean and refreshing it regularly is necessary.

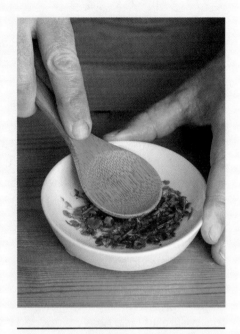

Basic Poultice Recipe

2–5 fresh herb leaves

1–3 teaspoons hot water

Dice the fresh herb leaves and place in a small bowl. Add enough hot water to mash and mix into a pastelike consistency. Apply to affected area for 15 to 20 minutes. Cover with a Band-Aid or sterile gauze wrap if you have to be on the go.

Salves

A salve, which is applied topically, can also be referred to as an ointment, a balm, an emollient, or sometimes a cream. Its base is typically beeswax, although many people have begun switching to vegan options such as candelilla wax and shea butter. By infusing herbs into oil and then adding the wax, you get a semisolid substance that can be spread onto the skin when and where it's needed. Used throughout history on animals and people, salves historically had bases of bear grease, lard, and other animal fats.

A salve is applied to soothe the body. Dabbing a bit of salve onto whatever is ailing you is an easy way to introduce herbs into your life. Most of us cannot get through a week without some small paper cut, hangnail, burn, or bug bite. Yes, all these will heal on their own, but why not offer yourself a touch of relief? Is a heavy workload causing you some muscle tension? Apply a bit of relief salve to relax the tension. Herbal medicine is just as much about learning to take the time to care for yourself as it is about healing specific symptoms.

Once you've decided which condition you're trying to remedy with a salve, you need to decide if you'd like the salve to be scented or not. Adding essential oils to the salve will help it smell good and also provide extra healing potential and a longer shelf life. Doing a bit of research regarding essential oils will really pay off in the end. With each salve recipe later in the book, I indicate specific essential oils that will complement the healing process. That being said, if you plan to use your salve quickly and prefer it to be unscented, that is fine too. Just keep it in a cool place for longevity.

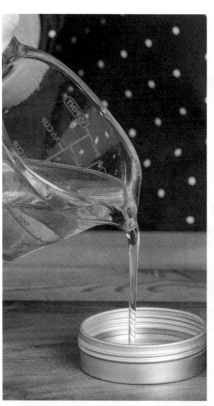
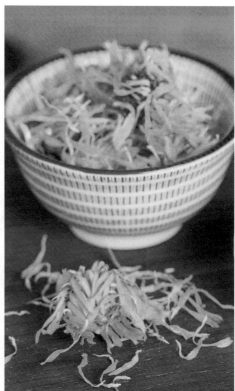
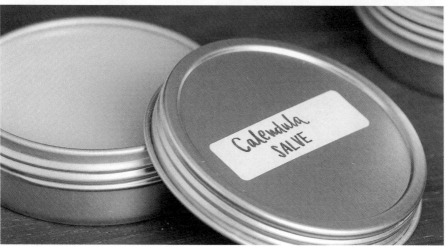

All you need in order to make a salve is a medicinal herbal oil, beeswax, and a container to put it in. It really is that simple. When using a salve, a little goes a long way but you always want to cover the area completely. Having a little bit sit on top of the injured area is just fine—it acts as a natural bandage.

Basic Salve Recipe

½ cup herbal oil

½ ounce beeswax

20 drops essential oil of your choice (optional)

Gently heat the oil, add the beeswax, and stir until melted. Add essential oil if you choose. Pour the salve into a jar. Let it cool completely before putting on the lid.

Sprays

Sprays are easy to create and use. Just a spritz here and a spritz there can quickly shift emotions, calm inflammation, soothe a cut, or transform the smell of a room.

Basic Spray Recipe

1–2 ounces distilled water

10–20 drops essential oil(s) or 1 ounce herbal tincture

Pour the water into a 2-ounce spray bottle and add your essential oil(s) or herbal tincture. Shake gently before spritzing.

Syrups

The base of any syrup is a strong herbal tea that has been simmered and reduced to create a concentrated brew. This is then combined with honey or sugar and voilà, you have herbal syrup. It's another example of the ease of making herbal medicines. If the medicine from an herb is water soluble, you can make an herbal syrup.

You may be familiar with elderberry syrup, as it hit the mainstream several years ago. High in antioxidants and with antiviral properties, it's a great addition to any household's medicine cabinet. And of course most of us have experienced cough syrup at some point in our lives. But syrups aren't just for colds and flus. You can also make headache syrup, mineral syrup, hair tonic syrup, and kids' tummy tamer syrup. The extra bonus is that herbal syrups typically taste delicious and are an easy way to get even the pickiest of palettes to try herbal medicine.

The question that typically arises here is: If I'm using leaves and flowers, won't the simmering hurt the final product? Honestly, I don't have an answer here. I often think of Susun Weed when I'm asked this question. In one conversation we had, we were discussing eating our greens verses taking vitamins and herbs to get our calcium. We agreed that eating greens is by far superior to getting the nutrient in other ways. I like to cook greens lightly, but Susun, like my mother, is big on cooking greens way down, reasoning that this allows for complete breakdown of the plant material so it can be readily assimilated in the body. I grew up with mushy vegetables, and once I began studying nutrition

I was thrilled to learn that light cooking kept many nutrients intact. So you can see my dilemma. To cook or not to cook down? There are good reasons either way; it just depends on what you're hoping to get. So for syrups, when you're trying to create a thick, concentrated base, cooking the herbs down on low heat makes sense to me.

Basic Syrup Recipe

4–6 cups water

1 ounce dried herbs

2–3 cups honey or sugar

Bring the water to a boil in a saucepan and add the herbs. Lower the heat and simmer with the lid on or ajar until the liquid is reduced by half. Double strain the herbs from the liquid. Pour the liquid into a measuring cup to measure, then pour back into a clean saucepan and add an equal amount of honey or raw cane sugar. Gently heat on low, continuously stirring until the honey or sugar has dissolved. Allow to cool then transfer into an amber bottle. Refrigerate if you've made a large batch.

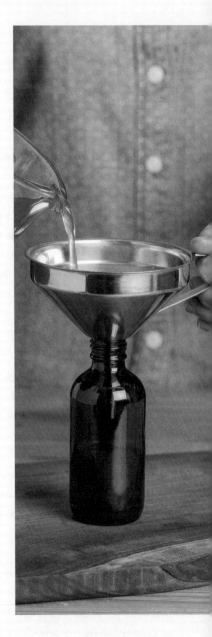

Tinctures

A tincture is a solution created by soaking an herb in alcohol to extract its healing properties, resulting in a medicine that can be taken by mouth. While tinctures can be made in mediums other than alcohol, such as vinegar or vegetable glycerin, alcohol is the most commonly used. The advantages of using alcohol are that it works with almost any plant (unlike vinegar or glycerin), you can formulate the optimal alcohol percentage in which a plant's constituents will extract (the plant's solubility range), and the alcohol base allows for sublingual transmission, meaning the medicine will bypass the digestive system and go more directly into the bloodstream—particularly helpful when medicine is needed to treat an acute situation. When I'm having menstrual cramps, for example, I take a tincture so it begins to work right away instead of taking a capsule and having to wait 40 minutes. A tincture definitely has an alcohol flavor, so if you cannot tolerate that, refer to the sidebar to see whether the herbs you'd like to use can be extracted with apple cider vinegar or vegetable glycerin.

To make a tincture, I recommend starting small. There is no need to create a quart of burdock tincture for yourself unless you want a lifetime supply or are planning to share it with your friends. Use 1- to 4-ounce jars to begin with. Start with making a simple, one-herb tincture. You can use either fresh or dried herbs when making a tincture, and for practicality's sake I'll only describe the folk tincture-making method in this book. If you are looking for other tincture-making options, please refer to my earlier book, *The Herbal Apothecary*.

Herbs that can be extracted with vinegar or glycerin

- burdock root
- chamomile flower
- cleavers leaf
- dandelion leaf and root
- echinacea root
- elderberries and elderflowers
- fennel seed
- ginger root
- goldenseal root
- hawthorn berries, leaf, and flower
- mugwort leaf
- mullein leaf
- nettle leaf and seed
- oat tops, leaf, and stem
- peppermint leaf
- Siberian ginseng root
- skullcap leaf and stem
- uva ursi leaf
- valerian root
- vitex berries

If using fresh leaves, flowers, roots, or bark, cut the material into small pieces before putting it into your extracting jar. Fill the jar halfway with your herb of choice (I often put in more for good measure). When using dried herbs, fill the jar a fifth to a third full. Then add vodka, filling the jar to the top, and close with a tight-fitting lid. Vodka's 40 to 50 percent alcohol by volume makes it a good fit for most herbs. The higher up the vodka is on the shelf at the liquor store, the better the quality, which equates with better taste. (Taste is hugely important to me as the better it tastes, the more likely I am to take it. When a tincture tastes like burning fuel, I tend to struggle with the desire to take it.) Next, label the jar with the name of the herb, today's date, and the date 4 weeks from now. Give it a good shake and set it somewhere where you'll remember to shake it daily. The shaking is important, as it agitates the plant material to break down and release the plant's constituents. Watch over the next 4 weeks as the color shifts and changes. This a favorite phase for me. I often feel very connected to the plant during this phase, as my intention is with it almost daily.

After the 4 weeks, strain the tincture twice through a fine-mesh sieve or a cheesecloth-lined colander to ensure all particulate matter is out. Store the tincture in a dark amber or blue dropper bottle with a proper name label and date. To maintain potency, tinctures are best kept out of direct sunlight, in a cool pantry or cupboard. While I don't believe in a shelf life for tinctures that have been stored properly, you can safely consider them viable for 3 to 5 years.

Sometimes I recommend using already prepared and purchased tinctures to make tincture blends. In these cases, the measurements are in milliliters to correspond to how purchased tinctures are packaged.

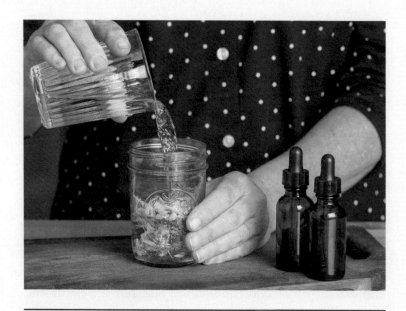

Basic Tincture Recipe

fresh or dried herb

vodka

If the herb is fresh, cut it into small pieces. Fill a 4-ounce jar a third full with the herb and fill to the top with vodka. Close tightly and shake well. Allow to macerate (to soften by soaking) for 4 weeks in a cool, dark place, shaking daily. Strain and transfer the liquid into a dark blue or amber dropper bottle for future use.

Washes

I use the term *herbal wash* to describe a single herb or a blend of herbs used to bathe, wash, or soak a part of the body. A great example is my eczema wash at Fettle. Eczema ranges in severity from mild to debilitating, but any form is uncomfortable. Itching, cracking of skin, dryness, and pain can all accompany this condition. Steeping a blend of cooling, anti-inflammatory, and emollient herbs and allowing the affected body part to soak in the cooled-down brew often provides much-needed relief.

I've successfully used washes for pink eye, cradle cap, and various other skin conditions. I also put sitz baths into this category. Sitz baths are an old nature-cure technique derived from the German *sitzbad*, meaning a bath (*bad*) in which one sits (*sitzen*). They are often used after labor to heal the vagina and perineum and are also helpful with hemorrhoid healing and relief. It is a deeper submersion of the bottom, pelvis, and hip regions. As you can imagine, the herbal wash targets the tissues in need, but it also works to gently move circulation and lymph channels in the area. While you can do a sitz bath in a shallow bathtub, you will find it difficult to get the herb-to-water ratio right. I prefer to use a plastic washbasin because you get the greatest surface area covered with a concentrated medicinal brew.

Even stronger than a medicinal-strength tea, an herbal wash is made with a recommended 6 tablespoons of herb per quart or 3 tablespoons per pint. I also suggest steeping the herbs for 1 or 2 hours before using the wash. You can steep overnight if you prefer and reheat if necessary. Soaking for 20 to 60 minutes is best.

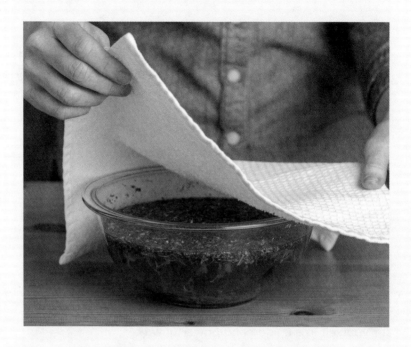

Basic Wash Recipe

6 tablespoons dried herb or herbal mixture

1 quart hot water

Pour the hot water over the herbs and close the container with a lid. Let steep 1 or 2 hours or overnight. Strain and pour the brew into a basin. Rewarm if necessary for treatment. Soak the affected body part 20 to 60 minutes.

Key Ingredients

Herbs for Day-to-Day Use

The herbs profiled here are those I recommend to create a beginner's library. These are good all-round, all-star herbs because they are readily available and generally considered safe for public consumption. As you read through the book, you will create your own list of herbs that call to you. Having a small, curated herbal medicinary in your home enables you to care for yourself in a unique and powerful way.

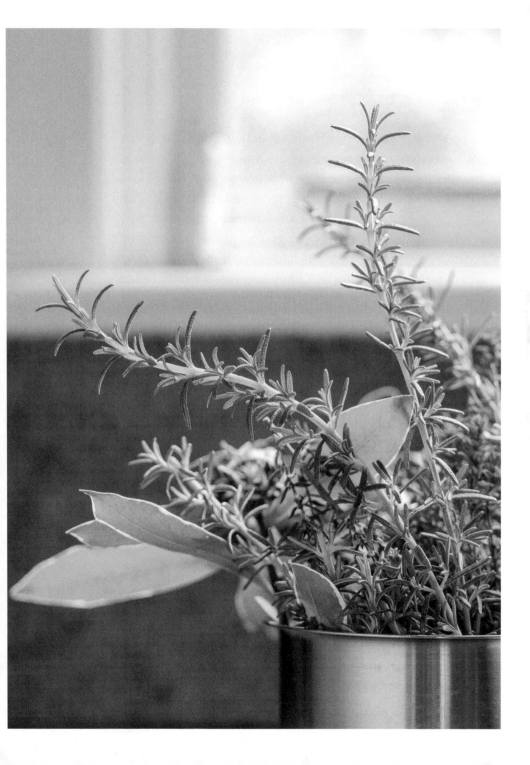

Where to Get Herbs

As you'll see, many herbs overlap in action, but not all herbs grow everywhere, hence the need to reference many options and then to learn which herbs grow in your region. You can always purchase herbs from reputable herb shops, but finding them in your local area is a fun adventure and gives new insight into the herbs. Growing your own medicinal herbs is also a rewarding experience and is more sustainable than collecting them from the wild. If you do the latter, it's called wildcrafting, and it's important to follow these rules:

- Ensure the plants have not been sprayed with pesticides.

- Ensure you are collecting the correct plant.

- Ensure the plant is not endangered from overcollecting. If it is, admire but do not collect.

- If harvesting, take only a quarter of the plant population found in the area. This ensures future generations of the plant will thrive.

- Never harvest bark from a live tree. Look for fallen branches to collect from.

- As a personal favor, I ask you to speak to the plant first before collecting. While plants are willing to share their medicine with us, it is kind to be grateful for it.

Ashwagandha

Withania somnifera
Parts used: roots

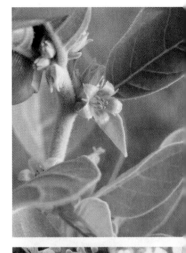

Usually in the immune defense department, this herb supports immune system health and also balances out the body, particularly the mood. I have seen ashwagandha alone uplift a patient's mood and affect after it has been taken consistently for 2 weeks. When the body feels strong and well, it is much easier to have a positive outlook.

Black cohosh

Actaea racemosa
(also *Cimicifuga racemosa*)
Parts used: rhizomes and roots

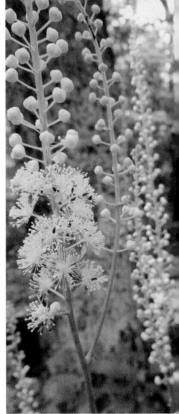

This herb, commonly thought of as a women's reproductive herb, has an amazing effect on calming the central nervous system. When someone's anxiety triggers the physical response of tremors, black cohosh should be included in the formula. I once had a patient who would begin to shake as if she were cold every time she became nervous or anxious, or thought about something worrisome. Using a nervine blend that included black cohosh made a significant improvement. As it is a smooth muscle relaxant, I often also use it to calm muscle tension.

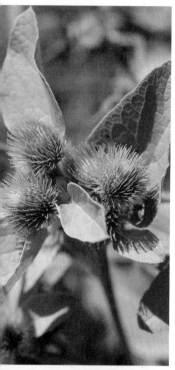

Burdock

Arctium lappa
Parts used: roots

Traditionally thought of as a liver herb, burdock root offers consistent support for the detoxification process and direct healing for the lining of the stomach and its function. The root is most often used, but the leaves create mild bile stimulation and are used as a wash for poison oak/ivy. I often use burdock root for those who need more grounding in their lives, those who are scattered by too much thought or responsibility, or those whose head is always in the clouds. If your energy is perpetually up and running or you tend to live outside of your body, burdock is a good choice. Be careful using it with those who already demonstrate a depressive nature.

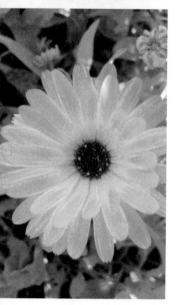

Calendula

Calendula officinalis
Parts used: flowers

Nature's healing flower, Calendula is known to pull tissues together to expedite healing. Antibacterial by nature, it is a great herb to keep areas free from infection while working to heal the wound. Used internally for gastritis, menstrual pain, fever, and recurring vomiting. The bright, beautiful flowers of calendula are always a hit with little ones. And when they learn that these flowers can help heal their cuts and scrapes, things get really exciting.

Catnip

Nepeta cataria

Parts used: leaves

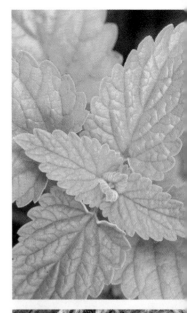

Not just for cats! This herb is one of the best for nervous stomach issues. When kids are young, they first learn about being in their bodies. What this means is identifying bodily sensations such as hunger, thirst, and needing to use the bathroom; then the identification of emotions begins. This is often when I see pediatric patients who complain of stomachaches. Kids are notorious for holding emotions in their tummies, and catnip is a great herbal ally to call upon in such times.

Celery

Apium graveolens

Parts used: seeds

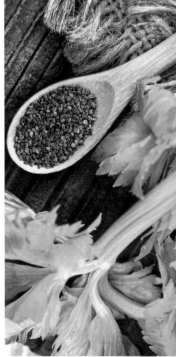

One of my go-to herbs for anxiety. I'd read about its ability to alleviate stress and particularly anxiety symptoms some years back and decided to give it a try with one of my patients, who couldn't stop her thoughts from spiraling out of control. The results were amazing. She immediately reported a sense of calm that she'd not felt in a long time.

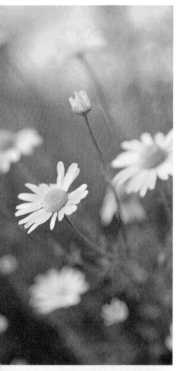

Chamomile

Matricaria chamomilla
Parts used: flowers

Most of us think of chamomile only for sleepy time teas, but this herb provides a lot of healing opportunity. It helps with stomach complaints, skin irritations, allergies, eye pain, menstrual irregularity, stress, hemorrhoids, toothaches, and lower back pain. This gentle flower is particularly helpful for children. Easing discomforts of the stomach and head, it can be used in teas, glycerin-based tinctures, and fomentations. It is my go-to with my little boy, who often gets angry with pain. As he is just a baby, he doesn't understand pain and it makes him very frustrated. When this occurs and he cannot be comforted by even his favorite things, using chamomile has proven very helpful.

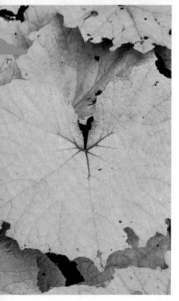

Coltsfoot

Tussilago farfara
Parts used: leaves

Coltsfoot is a respiratory herb that focuses on opening up breathing pathways to clear phlegm and constriction in the lungs. Antimicrobial by nature and soothing to the respiratory tract, it is excellent for dry cough and sore throat.

Comfrey

Symphytum officinale
Parts used: leaves

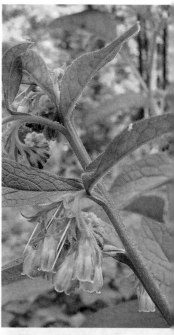

This herb grows tall and has what I refer to as fairy flowers along long stalks. With emollient, demulcent, and vulnerary properties, comfrey is a healing plant internally and externally. I use it for various skin afflictions and to soften the skin overall. Internally, it seems to help almost any chronic digestive problem, most likely due to its ability to soothe and coat the stomach and intestines with its protective constituents. Highly astringent, it can help to stop bleeding and excessive discharges from the body. The leaves can be applied to broken bones to help the healing process.

Cramp bark

Viburnum opulus
Parts used: bark

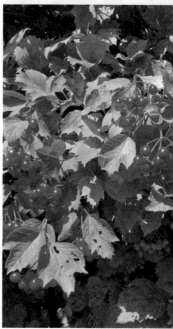

Cramp bark works to relax smooth muscle. It is often used for uterine cramping, but it will have effects on any smooth muscle of the body. A great addition to any reproductive blend.

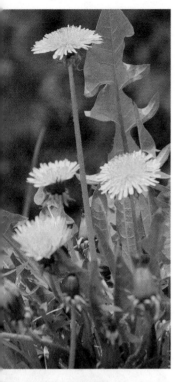

Dandelion
Taraxacum officinale

Parts used: leaves and roots

Both the leaf and root of dandelion offer wonderful medicine that can easily be incorporated into your daily diet. The leaves are only slightly bitter, and the root makes any stir fry a bit more lively. The root is considered an alterative herb, meaning it helps optimize the body's nutrient uptake and waste output and aids metabolism. This translates into helping the body clear toxins, so dandelion is often referred to as a blood cleanser. The leaves are diuretic and help the body maintain a healthy water balance. There have been reports of dandelion successfully reducing rheumatism, perhaps due to its ability to clear the body of built-up waste by-products.

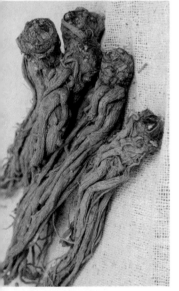

Dong quai
Angelica sinensis
Parts used: roots

Dong quai is a wonderful blood builder and blood mover often recommended for those who have pelvic stagnation, which leads to low menstrual flow or increased pain with menstruation. It is also a liver-supporting herb, so if you are inclined to believe the liver is involved in hormone imbalance, dong quai should be considered. You can make it into a tea or eat small amounts of the raw root each day. One of my teachers said to eat as much as the size of my pinky fingernail each day.

Echinacea

Echinacea purpurea
Parts used: roots

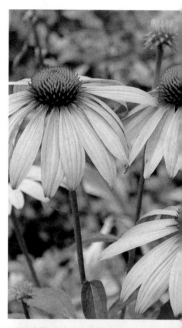

Everyone's favorite cold herb, echinacea is often misunderstood. It was one of the first herbs to hit the mainstream market, and the science had yet to catch up. Research shows that upon first use, echinacea activates white blood cells to increase and mobilize. This in turn stimulates the immune system, causing the natural defense cells to be on the lookout for foreign invaders. Taking echinacea continuously doesn't produce a continuous spike in natural defense; it's more a use-as-needed herb. If you're sitting next to a coworker who just went down with the flu, that's the time to take echinacea. Take it in small doses several times a day the first day or two of a cold or illness to boost your immune system's fighting powers, not continuously in hopes of building a stronger immune system. If you're unable to ward off a cold or flu after 2 days of taking echinacea, you must reexamine where the cold has settled and reassess your treatment going forward to minimize the duration of the illness.

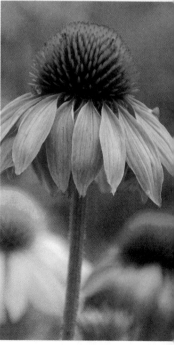

Echinacea can be used for so much more than just stimulating immune response. Use it topically for skin infections or internally for digestive bacterial infections. Some research shows that *Echinacea angustifolia* is helpful for cervical dysplasia. I often add echinacea to my pretravel tonics to protect me from the varying bacteria experienced on travel days. For babies and children, a glycerin drop formula makes it easy to dispense, and the glycerin's sweetness typically makes it widely accepted.

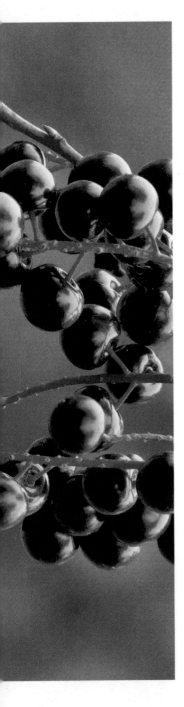

Elderberry

Sambucus nigra
Parts used: berries, flowers, and leaves

This plant with the little dark purple berry and the white elderflowers has really made the scene over the last few years. Elderberry syrup is a common recommendation for colds and flus, and it is said to be antiviral. Like most berries, elderberries are high in bioflavinoids and have antioxidant properties, helping to protect the body against free radicals and oxidative stress. An excellent research paper on elderberry created by the European Medicines Agency (Committee on Herbal Medicinal Products, "Assessment report on *Sambucus nigra* L., fructus," EMA/HMPC/44208/2012) demonstrates elderberry's effectiveness in relieving symptoms of influenza. I harvest it every year in fall and make a big batch of elderberry syrup, often adding splashes to all of our water bottles. I often add varying ingredients to my syrups such as echinacea root, reishi mushroom, cinnamon, cloves—really whatever I have in the medicine cabinet that may help in time of need for a cold or flu.

Elecampane

Inula helenium
Parts used: roots

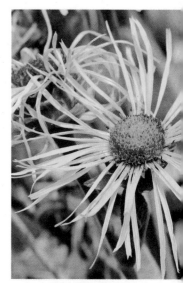

I first learned about elecampane from my mentor, Linda Quintana of Wonderland Teas and Spices in Bellingham, Washington. She taught me of its incredible healing potential for the lungs and often recommended it for lung rehabilitation. I use it when colds last too long and get into the deeper recesses of the bronchial tubes. It helps to pull phlegm up and out of the respiratory tract and also works to heal damaged lung tissue.

Eleuthero

Eleutherococcus senticosus
Parts used: roots

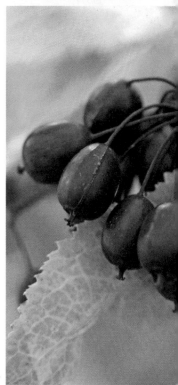

There are many ginseng-type herbs, and eleuthero is one of them. Eleuthero is known as Siberian ginseng, distinguishing it from Chinese ginseng and American ginseng. It is neutral when it comes to temperature, meaning it doesn't have the same heat-producing effects as these other ginsengs. Eleuthero is also much less stimulating and much more nourishing than the others. It is a tonic herb, used to balance immunity, mood, hormones, and stress.

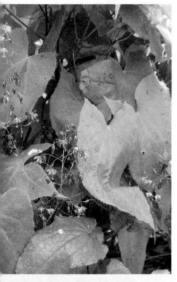

Epimedium

Epimedium sagittatum
Parts used: leaves

This herb is also known as horny goat weed because after several goats were seen eating it, their libidos seemed to increase. Now, I raised goats, and I'm not sure an increase in libido is possible with male goats, but we'll go with it. The active ingredient, icariin, has been shown to raise testosterone, and the herb overall has been shown to improve the circulation of testosterone and corticosterone and to raise nitric oxide levels in the body.

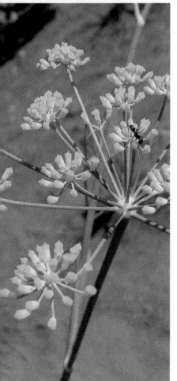

Fennel

Foeniculum vulgare
Parts used: seeds

Great for stomach upset, cramping, and lower bowel complaints. When a stomachache is obviously due to overeating, constipation, or illness, fennel can quickly provide relief from gas, colic, and intestinal tension. Fennel helps to loosen phlegm and congestion, making coughs more productive, and helps relieve the dry, hacking cough of bronchitis. It is used in many recipes to increase lactation. A decoction of the seeds has traditionally been used for generalized eye irritation.

Gentian

Gentiana lutea
Parts used: roots

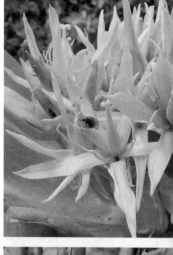

Digestive complaints often stem from what is eaten, stress, lack of proper digestive enzymes, medications, or eating too fast. The use of bitters—herbs that have a predominantly bitter taste, like gentian—is extremely helpful for almost any digestive complaint. Using bitters before a meal or at the onset of eating should help generate stomach acid to aid in the initial digestive process and support it through completion.

Ginger

Zingiber officinale
Parts used: roots

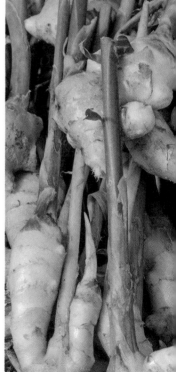

The anti-nausea herb, ginger is great for calming the stomach and relieving the sense of needing to vomit. This warming herb can be used throughout the body to reduce pain and cramping of the muscular kind. I recommend it when someone is experiencing a cold or flu but just can't quite mount the fever and immune response to kick it. Ginger will gently raise the fever to aid in burning out the infection invading the body. Ginger is also considered helpful to warm up the respiratory tract and release tension that may be restricting the ability to expel mucus.

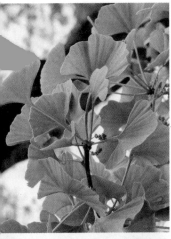

Ginkgo

Ginkgo biloba
Parts used: leaves

Ginkgo is commonly known for its memory-boosting powers. It increases oxygenation to the brain, allowing for clearer thinking. This action doesn't affect just the brain, though. It can help reduce PMS, increase libido, and decrease anxiety and depression, and it has even been reported to reduce headaches and migraines.

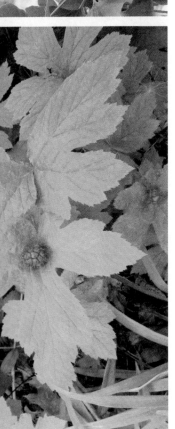

Goldenseal

Hydrastis canadensis
Parts used: roots

This amazing herb is unfortunately no longer abundant in the wild due to overharvesting, and because cultivating it is challenging, this herb has become very expensive. The double downside to this is that goldenseal's healing properties are hard to find in other herbs. Yes, other herbs contain berberine, which fights infection, but goldenseal's ability both to fight infection and to heal mucous membranes is an incredible combination. I use it internally and topically for various infections, and it is my go-to remedy for infections of the stomach and intestinal tract.

Hawthorn

Crataegus laevigata
Parts used: berries, leaves, and flowers

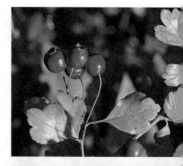

The berries, leaves, and flowers of hawthorn are all used in herbal medicine. The berries are specific to supporting the heart and cardiac function, whereas the leaves and flowers help circulation.

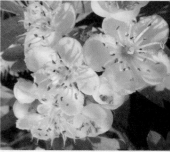

Hops

Humulus lupulus
Parts used: strobiles (flowers)

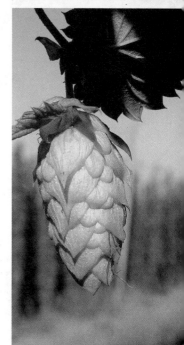

The flowers of the hop plant are called strobiles, and they have strong sedative effects. Working on both the nerves and the muscles, hops are helpful for many restless sleepers. Hops are bitter by nature and therefore work on the digestive system to varying degrees. I include hops in formulas for anxiety, sleep, digestive upset, and lactation. I find a little bit for the new mother helps her to relax into milk letdown and eases concerns over her ability to provide for her baby.

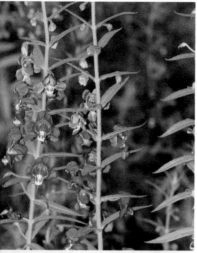

Hyssop

Hyssopus officinalis
Parts used: leaves

Sipped as a tea or taken as a tincture, hyssop has flu-fighting power, helping to ease muscle aches and respiratory congestion. It is known to increase circulation, which naturally mobilizes the immune system while also fighting infection. A gentle diaphoretic, it can also help to open up the pores to induce sweating when fever is present.

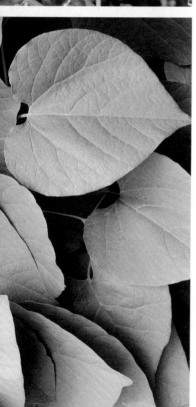

Kava Kava

Piper methysticum
Parts used: roots and rhizomes

A relatively new herb on the American market, kava has gained popularity as a sedative. It works by binding to various receptors in the brain, particularly the part of the brain known as the amygdala, which regulates feelings of fear and anxiety. It is also a muscle relaxant. Most people find deep relaxation in the use of kava.

Lavender

Lavendula species
Parts used: flowers

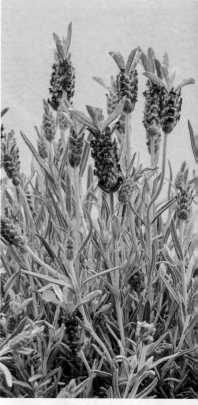

Lavender flowers are pretty, and their volatile oils offer a plethora of healing benefits, from tension and headache relief to soothing burns, expelling gas, and calming upset stomachs and unsettled emotions. They are antimicrobial, antibacterial, sedative, carminative, and anti-spasmodic in nature—excellent for relieving heat and healing skin. Using lavender flowers is one of my favorite ways to introduce children to herbs. I often teach them how to create little lavender sachets, and it's rare to find a child who doesn't appreciate the smell. My daughter's preschool teacher would put a drop of lavender oil on the children's palms for them to rub together and smell before nap time to calm the high energy of the classroom.

Lemon balm

Melissa officinalis
Parts used: leaves

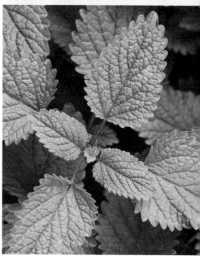

A gentle herb that calms overly excited nerves. Brew it up any time emotions have run high or stress is causing the heart to race or the stomach to churn. An antiviral, lemon balm has the ability to combat high viral loads. I often recommend it for dormant viral conditions such as shingles, herpes, and HPV. Its volatile oils also make it antimicrobial.

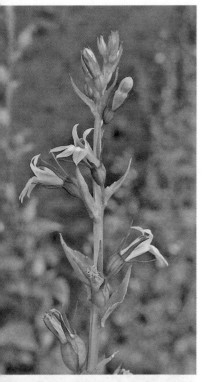

Lobelia

Lobelia inflata
Parts used: leaves and flowers

Lobelia is a field plant with emetic properties that, if accidentally consumed, causes purging. There is a story about a young boy who liked to play tricks on people and would give them lobelia. The odd thing was, while each person wasn't too happy about the experience, they all reported feeling amazing afterward. Lobelia has an incredible ability to purge the body, but it doesn't need to be in a violent way. Typically we use it to support the respiratory tract by opening and clearing the lungs. I've also used small amounts to increase sluggish circulation in order to warm up cold hands and feet. It has a very relaxing effect, and some use it to help induce sleep.

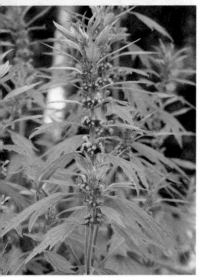

Motherwort

Leonurus cardiaca
Parts used: leaves, stems, and flowers

One of my favorites, this tall herb is thought to provide protection from negative energies when planted outside your home. Used as a heart medicine for centuries, it can calm and nourish the heart, and research shows it can decrease artery calcification. It also works on the endocrine system in supporting hormone balance. New research shows promising results from using it to treat Graves' disease.

Mugwort

Artemisia vulgaris
Parts used: leaves and stems

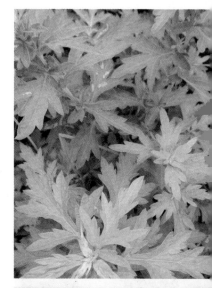

A sedative and liver tonic, mugwort is most commonly known to activate dream cycles. This is great if you are trying to remember and process your dreams, but not so great if you already have an active dream time, as it can leave one feeling quite tired in the morning from too much stimulation. Its liver actions help maintain hormone balance and seem to target the problem of menstrual irregularity.

Mullein

Verbascum thapsus
Parts used: flowers and leaves

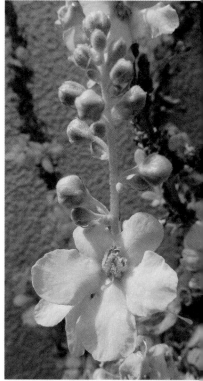

Mullein is a helpful herb to treat any cold. It moves mucus up and out while also calming respiratory irritation. The flowers of the mullein plant, which must be harvested and processed fresh, are an excellent tonic for ear pain and infection.

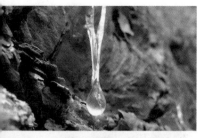

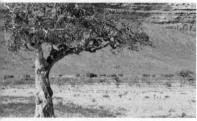

Myrrh
Commiphora myrrha
Parts used: oleo gum resin from the stem

Myrrh is a resin extracted from the bark of a small, thorny tree. Shown to have antibacterial, antifungal, antimicrobial, and antiseptic effects, myrrh is a great herb for colds and flus. I use it most for its drying capabilities, particularly for the drip-drip-drip of a runny nose. It can also open up nasal passageways, making sleep easier when there is congestion.

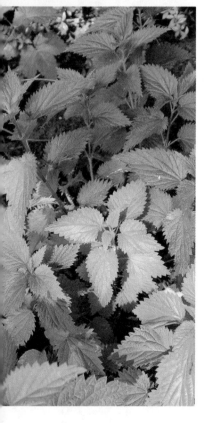

Nettle
Urtica dioica
Parts used: leaves, roots, and seeds

Nettle leaf, root, and seed are all used in herbal medicine and are anti-inflammatory. The seed is most commonly used in kidney blends, and both the leaf and root are used in prostate and male reproductive medicines. I've traditionally used nettle leaf anytime I've seen the need for a patient to get increased B vitamins and minerals. This can be due to generalize fatigued, laxity in ligaments, decreased breast milk, or debilitated functioning of one or more bodily systems. The leaves contain quercetin, which is helpful for seasonal allergy relief. Nettle leaf can also treat bladder weakness, and its astringency is called upon when it is used to treat excessive bleeding or leucorrhea. Also helpful in hair tonics.

Oatstraw

Avena sativa
Parts used: stems and leaves

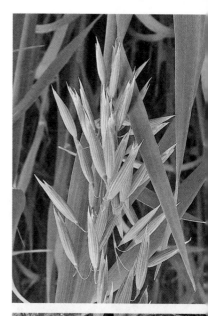

Oatstraw is one of those unassuming herbs that rarely gets talked about much anymore. Many people believe only the milky oat tops have medicinal value, but I prefer to use the oatstraw, believing it a better choice for long-term nourishing support. It is very gentle in action and packed with nutrients. This makes it helpful to anyone who has burned the candle at both ends and feels chronically run down and stressed.

Oregon grape

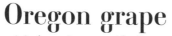

Mahonia aquifolium
Parts used: rhizomes and roots

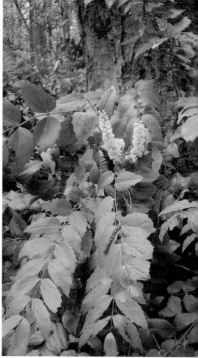

Oregon grape is an herb that works toward creating balance in the body. I've used it successfully for both diarrhea and constipation. It contains berberine, a powerful antibacterial agent. When something is off with the digestive system, I reach for Oregon grape first. It has traditionally been used for those who feel bloated, tired, toxic, and unconnected to their body.

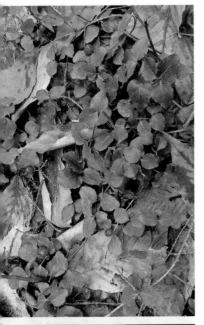

Partridge berry
Mitchella repens
Parts used: berries

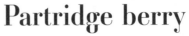

I find partridge berry a great herb for the overachieving woman—the woman who is stretched thin by all she has going on yet maintains it surprisingly well. Whether it shows or not, this does take a toll, and partridge berry does a great job of nourishing those who may be depleted. In combination it also calms and can be helpful for anxiety. A superior herb if dealing with infertility and menstrual irregularity, and very useful when bladder infections or inflammation arise.

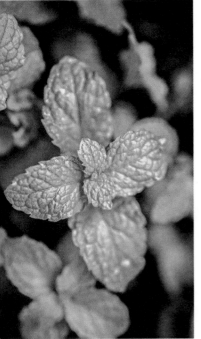

Peppermint
Mentha ×piperita
Parts used: leaves

A simple stimulant that can soothe the stomach, open the respiratory tract, and calm the central nervous system. Drink peppermint leaf tea to quell nausea, decrease muscle aches, and relieve the head of congestion. My favorite head cold remedy is a cup of peppermint tea, as I can breathe in the volatile oils that roll off the steam while I'm drinking it. These volatile oils work quickly and effectively. A few drops of essential oil to the temples or the nape of the neck have proven effective to calm tension headaches.

Pine

Pinus pinaster
Parts used: bark

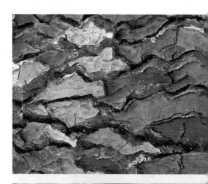

Pine bark is most often used for erectile dysfunction, but I use it for high cholesterol and to address sluggish circulation.

Plantain

Plantago major
Parts used: leaves, roots, and seeds

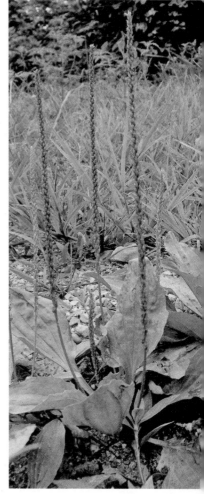

Plantain leaf is one of the herbs I consider a panacea. When in doubt, I try plantain. It soothes irritation, calms inflammation, draws out pain and infection, and heals mucous membranes and skin. It has also traditionally been used to soothe ulcers and toothaches, ease hoarseness of the voice, and rid the body of excess mucus. Teaching your child how to identify plantain at an early age will provide her or him with a lifetime of yellow jacket sting relief. Stings hurt, and the quicker you can put something helpful on them, the better. Finding a few leaves, chewing them up, and spitting them onto the sting is not only super fun for kids, it also distracts them and makes them proactive in helping themselves. The best part? It relieves the pain.

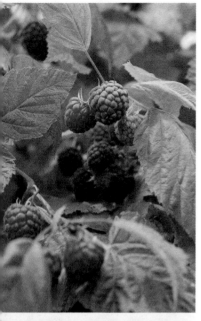

Raspberry
Rubus idaeus
Parts used: leaves

In women's health, raspberry (also commonly called red raspberry) is most often considered a nourishing tonic during pregnancy to prepare the uterus for delivery. Raspberry is also a superior gastrointestinal herb and used often for diarrhea and irritable bowel syndrome. Its astringent nature and high nutrient content make it very supportive to the physical body. It aids in fever management, and I often add it to my cold and flu teas due to its high vitamin C content.

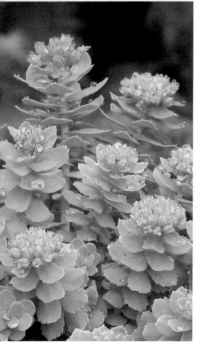

Rhodiola
Rhodiola rosea
Parts used: roots and bark

This is one of two adaptogen herbs (schisandra is the other) that are superior at supporting the adrenal glands and regulating the cortisol stress response. Both work to balance the function of the adrenals and return the body to normal cortisol release when someone has been living in a constant stress response cycle. When a patient reports chronic stress with symptoms of anxiety or insomnia, I typically include one of these herbs to provide support.

Rose

Rosa species
Parts used: petals and hips

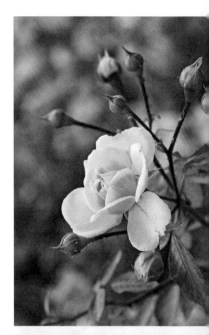

Roses seem to radiate peace. Just looking at one can evoke a sense of calm in my body, and the scent has an intoxicating effect upon my brain. While using roses in this way provides emotional healing, using them internally helps to stop bleeding. Rose petals were traditionally used for internal pains of the body—including headaches, tooth pain, sore throat, and stomach upset—for irritations of the respiratory tract, and for chronic, unproductive coughs.

Rosemary

Rosmarinus officinalis
Parts used: leaves

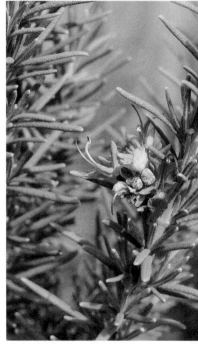

A stimulating herb, rosemary wakes us up and gets the brain juices flowing. It is often included in memory blends to stimulate cognitive function. I also add it in smaller quantities to dream blends to help people remember their dreams. Rosemary can be used to treat respiratory infections that present with excessive mucus and a wet cough. Its stimulating nature can also warm the skin and extremities by moving the blood. It was traditionally used to raise low blood pressure and stimulate circulation, so use it with caution if you are on medications for related

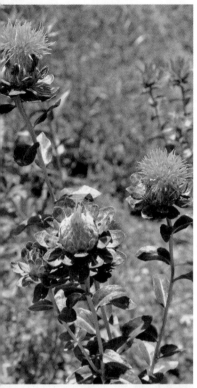

conditions. High in volatile oils, rosemary is an herb to plant along the pathway to your front door to purify guests before they enter.

Safflower

Carthamus tinctorius
Parts used: flowers

Although it does have blood-thinning properties, the delicate safflower is in my opinion an extremely underutilized herb. It has a tendency to travel to small spaces in the body, and it is exactly these small spaces where waste can accumulate. Safflower gently pushes out toxic build-up and decreases the potential for long-term damage to such areas as the joints and arteries. It is supportive in lowering cholesterol and blood pressure, and I use it to prevent blood clots.

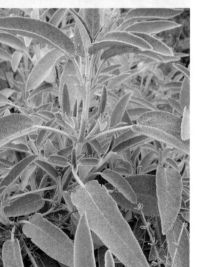

Sage

Salvia officinalis
Parts used: leaves

Almost any sore throat will benefit from sage leaf tea. Its soothing effects work to calm inflammation, and it is antibacterial and antiseptic. Drink it for systemic effects and gargle for target treatment to the throat. A great addition to any cold tea blend, it will work to break up congestion and relieve the discomforts of colds.

Saw palmetto

Serenoa repens
Parts used: berries

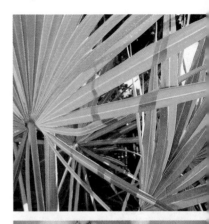

Saw palmetto is the most commonly pre-scribed herb for male prostate problems. It works to balance hormones of the reproductive system and seems to normalize the functioning of the prostate.

Schisandra

Schisandra chinensis
Parts used: berries

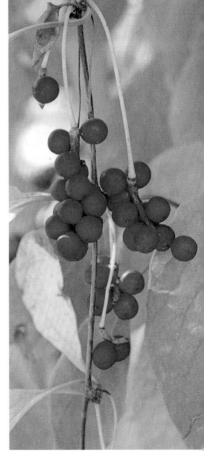

This is one of two adaptogen herbs (rhodiola is the other) that are superior at supporting the adrenal glands and regulating the cortisol stress response. Both work to balance the function of the adrenals and return the body to normal cortisol release when someone has been living in a constant stress response cycle. When a patient reports chronic stress with symptoms of anxiety or insomnia, I typically include one of these herbs to provide support.

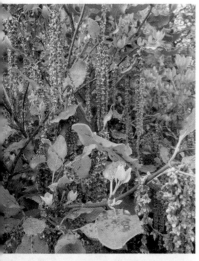

Silk tassel
Garrya eliptica
Parts used: leaves

Another wonderful herb that comes to the rescue when menstrual cramping is on the rise, silk tassel is a strong antispasmodic. If you are experiencing gastrointestinal cramping with bowel upset, silk tassel will work wonders in relieving you of the discomforts. It is extremely bitter and can be used as a quinine substitute.

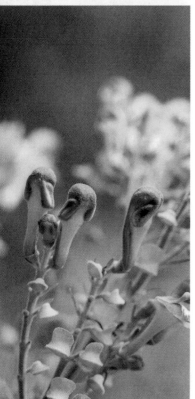

Skullcap
Scutellaria lateriflora
Parts used: leaves

A superior nutritive nervine that works to calm the nerves and give resilience. When we do too much in our lives, we tend to become depleted, and our stress centers become overactive. This can lead to excessive thinking and an inability to calm ourselves. Skullcap works to quiet the mind and clarify thoughts. Skullcap is also helpful to treat pain that inhibits sleep and for insomnia itself.

St. John's wort

Hypericum perforatum
Parts used: leaves and flowers

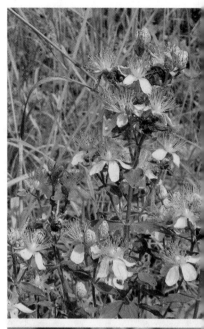

St. John's wort got its name from its traditional flowering and harvesting day—St. John's Day, June 24. Traditionally used for nerve pain and irritation, St. John's wort is an herb I've given to those suffering from neuralgia, neuropathy, and exposed nerve sensitivities. These days the research on St. John's wort is focused on its antidepressent effects, and I often add it to tea blends for this purpose. My patients like the subtle effect it seems to create, gently lifting the mood.

Tribulus

Tribulus terrestris
Parts used: fruit

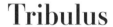

Also known as puncturevine, this low-growing plant with a prickly-looking thorn has been proven to raise testosterone levels. This improves libido and stamina, and many men report an increase in their sense of vitality.

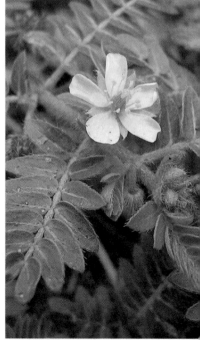

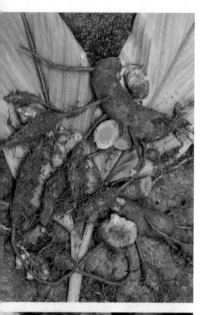

Turmeric

Curcuma longa
Parts used: roots

More and more research is coming out regarding the anti-inflammatory properties of turmeric. By adding turmeric to your diet, you can make your food into powerful medicine. Used for arthritis, rheumatism, and aches and pains, turmeric has the ability to move the blood and warm the tissues. Considered a blood purifier, turmeric can remove toxins from the blood and reduce the accumulation of metabolic by-products.

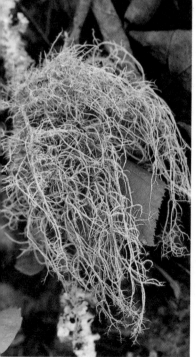

Usnea

Usnea barbata
Parts used: whole plant

Usnea is a type of lichen that can be seen throughout the forests of the Pacific Northwest, looking like witches' hair falling from the tree branches. Several lichens look similar, and proper identification is important. Usnea is a must-have for the immune defense medicine cabinet. Stephen Buhner's book *Herbal Antibiotics* discusses its antibiotic properties, and I often use it when I suspect a bacterial infection such as strep throat or when the flu comes on quickly with a high fever. Usnea needs to be cut up finely with scissors before being used in teas and tinctures.

Vervain

Verbena officinalis

Parts used: leaves

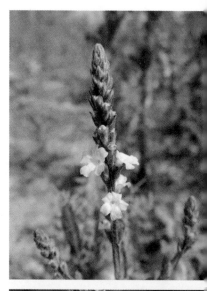

When anxious feelings pervade, particularly when one questions one's worth, I reach for vervain, a true nervine. It is calming and works as a tonic to both the central nervous and reproductive systems. Vervain can increase breast milk and quell dysmenorrhea when taken as a long-term tonic. Vervain may be the right choice for tension or menstrual headache relief as well.

Vitex

Vitex agnus-castus

Parts used: seeds and berries

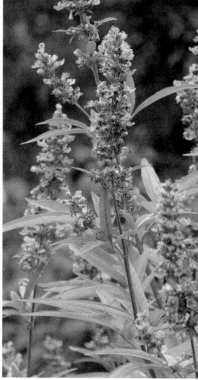

In ancient Greece, this herb was associated with chastity. Given to all maidens before marriage rites, it was also considered a fertility booster. It's an adaptogen by nature, meaning it helps create balance—whatever is low it raises, and whatever is high it lowers. Typically estrogen is dominant, so vitex works to lower it and to raise progesterone. It's often used for absence of menses, irregular menses, and other hormonal troubles such as acne, but it requires patience and consistent dosing. Those with polycystic ovary syndrome (PCOS) need to consult with their natural health care provider before using vitex, as not all PCOS patients will benefit from the herb.

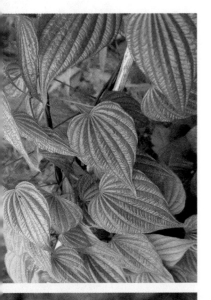

Wild yam
Dioscorea villosa
Parts used: roots

A root with estrogen-driving properties, wild yam is helpful when you are experiencing hormonal imbalance and it is causing vaginal dryness, PMS, bone loss, and/or decreased libido. Wild yam also has powerful antispasmodic and anti-inflammatory properties. A good herb to consider when joint pain is present or if gastrointestinal cramping is causing discomfort.

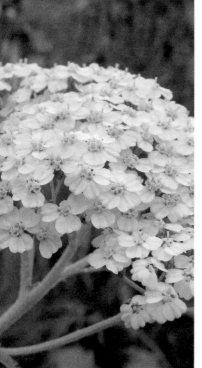

Yarrow
Achillea millefolium
Parts used: flowers, leaves, and stems

Yarrow is a gentle fever reducer and a powerful hemostatic. It is readily used for many different skin conditions, including bruising, wounds, bleeding, and pain; and for hot, stagnant conditions where blood is not moving well, including in the digestive tract, the circulatory system, and the reproductive system. When a cold and or fever strikes my kids and they are obviously ill (wanting to lie down), a small cup or even a few teaspoons of yarrow tea can alleviate the discomforts of fever, promote gentle sweating, stimulate the immune system, and improve the mood.

Yellow dock

Rumex crispus

Parts used: roots

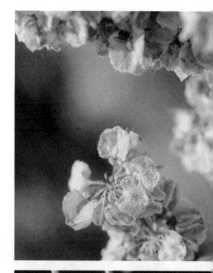

This herb is helpful for hormone regulation through supporting the liver and is often recommended when assimilation of iron is a problem. It is often used in women's reproductive formulas. Yellow dock was traditionally used to treat swollen, painful, and itchy skin. It is also helpful for lower digestive complaints where food feels like it isn't going anywhere.

Yohimbe

Pausinystalia johimbe

Parts used: bark

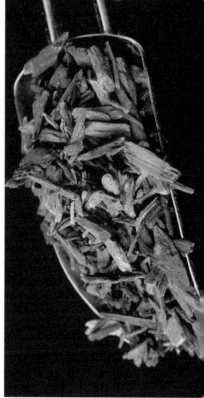

Yohimbe contains a chemical called yohimbine that can increase blood flow and nerve impulses to the penis. It is most commonly used as needed to treat erectile dysfunction and decreased libido.

Recipes for Immune Defense

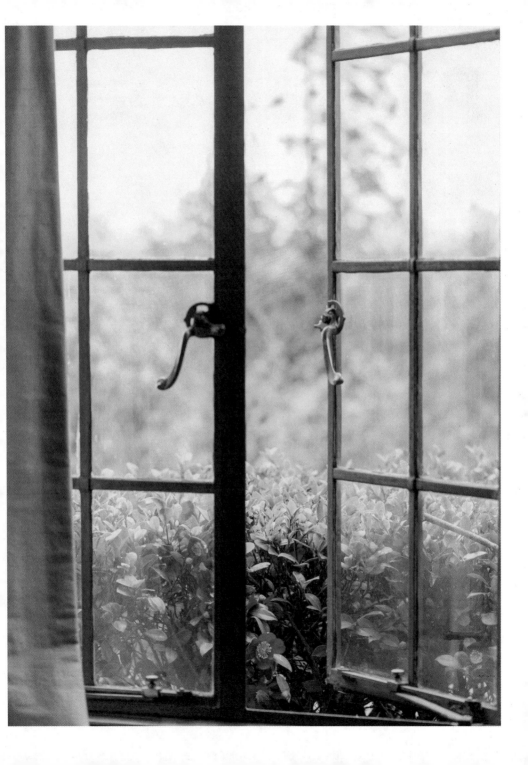

Dr. JJ's Tips
for When You Fall Ill

- Skip work, school, and events. You need to rest, and you have a responsibility to not expose others to your illness.

- At the onset of a cold or flu, take echinacea tincture, 1 dropperful every 3 hours for 1 or 2 days.

- Rest. I cannot overstate the value of rest when sick. Allowing the body to shut down and take care of what is ailing it makes a big difference. This doesn't mean staying home from work but being on the computer all day. It means lying in bed and trying to sleep as much as possible.

- Try a castor oil pack. The simple nature cure of a castor oil pack can mobilize the immune system to fight infection. Rub 2 tablespoons castor oil over the abdomen. Cover with a cotton towel and then a hot water bottle or heating pad. Relax for 30 to 45 minutes, or leave on overnight.

In this section, you'll find recipes to address immune system challenges you might encounter. Again, these recipes are not to replace professional care if you encounter serious health concerns. They are meant to reunite you with the knowledge of how to care for yourself. I hope they help you to reclaim the confidence to give your body what it needs during times of discomfort.

At the first sign of something coming on, do something about it. There are plenty of approaches to choose from, but be proactive. If you notice your coworker coughing all over the place, protect yourself with a few drops of Guard's-Up Tincture. If you're getting ready to travel, dose up before getting on an airplane, because once the door is shut we are all susceptible to whatever has come onboard. Same with the commuter bus or train. Rubbing a few drops of rosemary or lavender essential oil onto your hands and chest helps to block anything floating around.

Should you fall ill, I beg you to take gentle care of yourself. If it's safe for them to do so, let your partner, parent, or—if they're old enough—kids help you. Our society is so bad at asking for help, yet all most of us want is to care and be cared for. Please, break the cycle and teach others how to do so by accepting care in your own life.

COVID-19

As I write this, we still have a lot to learn about COVID-19. But here is what we have learned so far. In the body, SARS-CoV-2, the new coronavirus that causes COVID-19, attacks ACE2, a regulatory enzyme that sits on the outer surface of cells in such organs as the lungs, heart, kidney, liver, and intestines. When the virus enters the body, it attacks the ACE2 sites and damages them, creating an entry point. When coronavirus enters the cell, a reaction occurs almost instantly, resulting in the body's natural response in the form of an inflammatory cascade, which results in huge cytokine migration. Cytokines usually help the body fight infection, but an uncontrolled level can result in dangerous symptoms, including autoantibody production (when your antibodies attack healthy cells), hypoxia (oxygen deprivation), and endothelial (blood vessel lining) damage. Herbs that help protect ACE2 receptors include licorice, elder, Chinese skullcap, and horse chestnut. Cordyceps and rhodiola can help inhibit an autoantibody response, and rhodiola also helps diminish hypoxia.

Various studies have explored the remarkable ability of boneset and elecampane to boost resistance to various bacteria and viral strains. One study showed that boneset inhibited viral attachment of influenza A. While every virus is different, this study should make us curious about how boneset may help protect against other viruses. The symptom-relieving actions of boneset for fever, body aches, and chills make it a great consideration when combating any type of flu invasion. Elecampane is one of my favorite choices for a respiratory system in distress. I've seen it work wonders on stuck phlegm in the lower recesses of the lungs and for coughs that are due to infection or allergies.

As the first line of defense in the respiratory tract, cilia do their best to keep invaders out. Ensuring they are healthy and intact is an important way to keep immunity up. Herbs to protect the cilia include Oregon grape, cordyceps, and olive leaf.

The lymphatic system and spleen help protect the body in many ways, including creating and transporting infection-fighting white blood cells. Herbs to support them include poke, cleavers, dan shen, and Chinese skullcap.

Allergies

The key to allergy relief is to decrease histamine release and soothe mucous membranes, which aids in relieving symptoms.

My poor husband has suffered hay-fever allergies his entire life. While I look forward to spring, summer, and early fall, my husband has a level of hesitation about welcoming the changes of the seasons due to his suffering. I celebrate the smell of freshly cut grass, but he wears a bandana to mow the lawn. I am constantly pushing remedies on him, and when he takes them he has a break from the allergic cough, runny nose, red eyes, and sneezing.

Allergy-Tamer Capsules

½ ounce nettle leaf powder

½ ounce calendula flower powder

½ ounce fennel seed powder

½ ounce yerba santa leaf powder

Mix the powders in a bowl and fill 200 empty capsules. Take 2 capsules twice per day.

Allergy-Tamer Tea

1 ½ ounces rose hips

1 ounce yerba santa leaf

½ ounce nettle leaf

½ ounce orange peel

½ ounce lemongrass

Mix the herbs in a bowl and store in a glass jar. Use 4 to 5 tablespoons to make 1-quart batches. Drink 2 to 3 cups per day for 6 to 8 weeks, or as needed.

Neti pot formula
for allergies

When you experience allergies, it is very important to care for your respiratory system and the mucous membranes that are under attack. One of the best ways to do this is to use a neti pot twice a day. I can attest to their positive results in clearing out particles that have been inhaled that are causing problems. By rinsing these from your nasal system, you are decreasing the overall irritant load. Try adding 1 dropper of wild cherry bark tincture to your neti pot along with the usual salt (follow the instructions that come with the pot). Wild cherry bark is known to help decrease histamine reactions in the body.

Hay-Fever Eyewash

1 ounce nettle leaf

1 ounce calendula flower

1 ounce chickweed leaf

1 ounce eyebright leaf

Mix the herbs in a bowl and store in a glass jar. When needed, put 5 tablespoons in a pint jar and pour boiling water over the herbs to fill the jar. Let steep 1 hour and then strain. You can keep the herbs to reuse. Soak a cotton cloth in the infusion and douse the eye, inside and out, with it. Repeat 4 to 6 times a day.

Hay-Fever Tea

1 ounce chamomile flower (purchased from a reputable source so that cross-contamination with ragweed is not an issue)

1 ounce peppermint leaf

½ ounce elderflower

½ ounce nettle leaf

Mix the herbs in a bowl and store in a glass jar. Make tea by the cup. Steep 1 or 2 teaspoons in 10 ounces of hot water, covered, for 10 minutes. Drink as needed or 3 cups a day during days of heightened pollen count.

Antiviral Treatments

Is it a bacteria or a virus? Generally, viruses come on slowly, create low fevers, and cause lingering symptoms, while bacterial infections come on more quickly, create higher fevers, and cause stronger first symptoms. The common cold, the flu, and a generalized sore throat are most often viral, whereas bronchitis, ear infections, strep throat, and whooping cough are most often bacterial. Bacterial infections often debilitate us. There is often no hiding the fact that we are sick. This typically forces us to cease daily routines and rest. Viral infections, on the other hand, can go on and on. This compromises the immune system, making it vulnerable to the next cold that comes along. Have you ever had one cold and been almost over it only to fall ill again? Although the symptoms of viral colds are often tolerable, we should still be aware that our body is weakened. Continuing on with our regular routine can further compromise the healing process and our health. Reach for an herbal remedy the next time a virus comes on.

Antiviral Tea

Whether you're up against the latest viral cold on the block or a reacquaintance with a cold sore or shingles, this tea can help you fight it off.

2 ounces lemon balm leaf

1 ounce elderberry

¼ ounce lomatium root

¼ ounce usnea

¼ ounce yarrow flower

¼ ounce ginger root

Mix the herbs in a bowl and store in a glass jar. Steep 4 to 5 tablespoons in a quart jar and drink 3 cups a day.

Antiviral Tincture

Sometimes bypassing the digestive system is necessary when sick. Having direct entry through tissues can give more support to the nerves as well.

2 tablespoons echinacea root

2 tablespoons lomatium root

1 tablespoon goldenseal root

1 tablespoon usnea

1 tablespoon licorice root

1 pint vodka

Put the herbs in a 1-pint glass jar and fill to the top with vodka. Close the lid tightly and shake well. Store in a cupboard or pantry for 3 weeks, shaking daily. Strain and transfer to your container of choice. Take 1 dropperful twice daily if experiencing high stress, or take 2 dropperfuls 3 to 4 times a day during an acute viral infection. Do not use long term.

Antiviral Cream

This formula is based on one originally created by herbalist Kerry Bone. I used to make it often for patients and always had positive results. Typically used for a herpes outbreak, it may also be helpful for shingles and the irritation of measles and chicken pox.

4 ounces previously prepared lemon balm tincture

1 ounce St. John's wort leaf and flower

1 ounce lomatium root

4 cups water

8 ounces cocoa butter

8 ounces shea butter

2 ounces beeswax

Simmer the lemon balm tincture on the stove top on low until it is reduced by half. In a separate pan, combine the St. John's wort, the lomatium, and the water. Simmer covered on low until reduced by half and then strain. Add the reduced lemon balm tincture to the St. John's wort–lomatium extract and allow to cool slightly. In the meantime, melt the oils together in a separate pan over low heat. Once they are the same temperature, mix the extract into the oils until they emulsify then transfer to your container of choice. Apply this cream at the first tingle of a herpes outbreak and thereafter several times a day. Always use a clean Q-tip and never double dip.

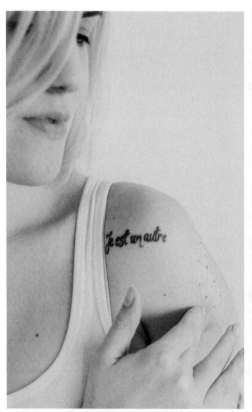

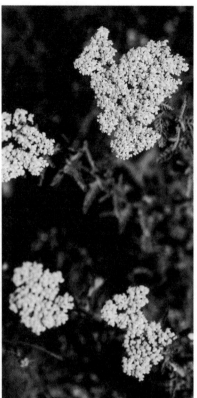

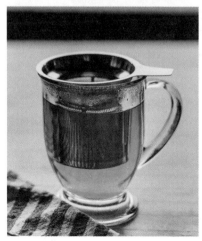

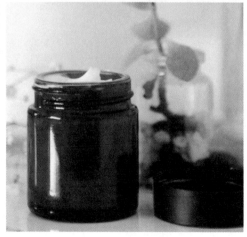

Breathing

The inability to breathe is a scary and life-threatening situation. These formulas are by no means an attempt to replace medications necessary to control asthma or other respiratory distress, but my experience has shown they can lead to a decrease in the frequency and quantity of medications required.

Better-Breathing Tincture

1 ½ ounces yerba santa leaf

1 ¼ ounces black cohosh root

1 ounce cramp bark

¼ ounce lobelia leaf

¹⁄₁₆ ounce cayenne powder

4 ounces vodka

Place all the herbs in a 4-ounce glass jar. Cover with vodka to a depth of 1 to 2 inches. Close and shake well. Put in a cool, dark place like a cupboard or pantry for 3 weeks, shaking every day. Strain and transfer to a dropper bottle. Take 2 dropperfuls twice daily or as needed, not to exceed six doses per day.

Bronchitis

The hacking of bronchitis is distinct and hard to miss. Bronchitis can start as a cold that then drops down into the chest and settles, or it can start as a respiratory infection right off the bat. Whichever way it starts, the end result is inflammation and irritation of the lining of the bronchial tubes, which bring air into the lungs. Each time you breathe in, the lining is irritated and coughing ensues. Smokers and those whose respiratory systems are compromised are the most vulnerable. Bronchitis often leaves one feeling wiped out. Symptoms include shortness of breath, a rattling or dry cough, phlegm production, and wheezing—upper respiratory symptoms can be present at the same time. Although typically bacterial, the cough can last for weeks as the respiratory system works to decrease inflammation and heal from the infection.

Acute-Bronchitis Tincture

2 teaspoons elecampane root

½ teaspoon myrrh resin

½ teaspoon cinnamon bark

½ teaspoon mullein leaf

½ teaspoon safflower flower

2 ounces vodka

Put the herbs in a 2-ounce jar and add vodka to fill. Close tightly and shake well. Keep in a pantry or cupboard for 3 weeks, shaking every day. Strain and transfer to a 2-ounce dropper bottle. Take 2 dropperfuls 3 to 4 times a day for 2 weeks.

Bronchitis-Soothing Syrup

1 ounce elecampane root

½ ounce borage leaf

¼ ounce coltsfoot leaf

¼ ounce cinnamon bark

8 cups water

3 cups cane sugar or honey

¼ cup apple cider vinegar

Put the herbs in a saucepan with the water. Bring to a boil and reduce by half over medium-low heat. Strain the herbs out and put the brew back into the pan. Add sugar or honey and gently heat to mix if necessary, stirring continuously. Turn off the heat, add the apple cider vinegar, and allow to cool. Transfer to your container of choice and store in the refrigerator. Take 1 teaspoon 3 to 4 times a day.

Bronchitis-Calming Tea

1 ounce peppermint leaf

¾ ounce hyssop leaf

¾ ounce elecampane root

½ ounce thyme leaf

½ ounce marshmallow root

¼ ounce sage leaf

¼ ounce vervain leaf

Mix the herbs in a bowl and store in a glass jar. Simmer 3 table-spoons over low heat in 20 ounces of water, covered, for 10 minutes. Turn off the heat, add 2 teaspoons, cover, allow to steep for 10 minutes, then strain. You should have 18 ounces, which you can divide into 3 cups of 6 ounces each. Drink hot. When suffering from acute symptoms, drink 2 to 4 cups a day.

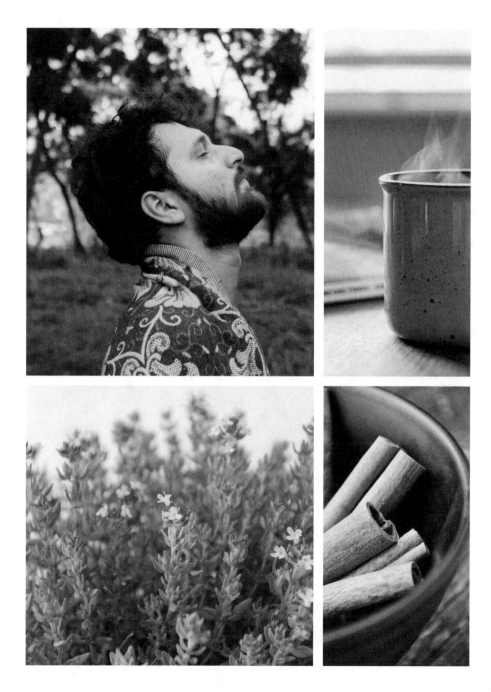

Catarrh

Catarrh is the medical term for the presence of excessive mucus or phlegm in the nose and throat. Inflammation of the mucous membranes is also present. Sometimes our nose turns into a leaky faucet with no other symptoms present. Other times we are so congested with a cold that breathing through our nose is next to impossible. Catarrh can also lead to a cough as the phlegm slides down the back of the throat and irritates the mucous membranes. Breaking up the phlegm, drawing it out, and soothing inflammation are what these herbs do best. Stay overly hydrated during these times as it helps to dilute the mucus.

Open-Up Tincture

Great for when excessive mucus has you blocked in your head or chest.

2 teaspoons myrrh resin

1 teaspoon sumac bark

½ teaspoon angelica root

½ teaspoon goldenseal root

2 ounces vodka

Put the herbs in a 2-ounce jar and add vodka to fill. Close tightly and shake well. Keep in a pantry or cupboard for 3 weeks, shaking every day. Strain and transfer to a 2-ounce dropper bottle. Take 1 dropperful 3 times a day until symptoms subside.

Catarrh-Dispersing Tea

1 ¼ ounces peppermint leaf

1 ounce bayberry

1 ounce coltsfoot leaf

½ ounce comfrey leaf

¼ ounce ginger root

Mix the herbs in a bowl and store in a glass jar. Make tea by the cup. Steep 1 or 2 teaspoons in 10 ounces of hot water, covered, for 10 minutes. Drink hot, 4 cups a day until symptoms subside.

Diffuser Blend for Catarrh

5 milliliters spikenard essential oil

3 milliliters cedarwood essential oil

2 milliliters benzoin essential oil

Mix the oils in a 10-milliliter essential oil bottle. Add 5 drops to your diffuser at bedtime.

Chest Colds

Chest colds range from simple respiratory congestion to severe compromise. Symptoms often include
cough, wheezing, sore throat, runny nose, phlegm
production, tight chest, fever, and fatigue. Whenever
your primary breathing system is compromised,
fatigue is inevitable. Chest colds can be bacterial
or viral, and the cough can vary from wet to dry to
sticky. You should always treat a cough, as the longer
it lasts the greater opportunity it has to take a turn
for the worse. See the separate "Coughs" section to
get specific with your cough for best treatment. And
if you want to dive deeper into the respiratory system, you'll find even more detailed information in my
book *The Herbal Apothecary*.

Chest-Cold Tea

1 ounce mullein leaf

1 ounce elecampane root

¾ ounce rosehips

½ ounce elderflower

½ ounce elderberry

¼ ounce juniper berry

Mix the herbs in a bowl and store in a glass jar. Make tea by the cup. Steep 1 or 2 teaspoons in 10 ounces of hot water, covered, for 10 minutes. You can also steep 4 to 5 tablespoons in a quart jar, and then you have a day's worth of tea ready to go. Drink hot, 4 cups a day until symptoms subside.

Chest-Cold Tincture

1 teaspoon usnea, pulverized or cut up

1 teaspoon yarrow flower

1 teaspoon ashwagandha root

½ teaspoon white horehound leaf

½ teaspoon marshmallow root

Put the herbs in a 2-ounce jar and add vodka to fill. Close tightly and shake well. Keep in a pantry or cupboard for 3 weeks, shaking every day. Strain and transfer to a 2-ounce dropper bottle. Take 1 to 2 dropperfuls 4 times a day.

Chest-Cold Salve

1 tablespoon hyssop leaf

1 tablespoon licorice root

1 tablespoon ginger root

1 teaspoon lobelia leaf and flower

¾ cup olive oil

½ ounce beeswax

50 drops eucalyptus citriodora essential oil

Put the herbs in a glass baking dish and cover with olive oil to a depth of 1 or 2 inches. Bake at 170 degrees F for 4 hours. Allow to cool and then strain. Pour the oil into a saucepan and add the beeswax. Gently heat until the beeswax is melted. Add the essential oil and pour into a jar. Apply to chest, neck, and upper back.

Diffuser Blend for Chest Colds

4 milliliters juniper essential oil

4 milliliters lemon essential oil

2 milliliters clove essential oil

Mix the oils in a 10-milliliter essential oil bottle. Add 5 drops to your diffuser at bedtime.

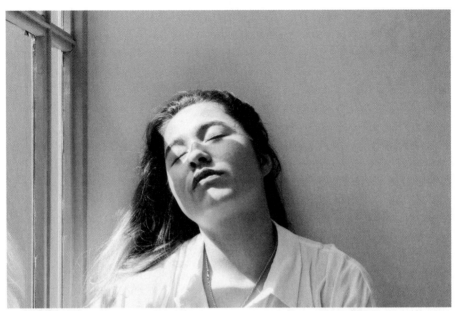

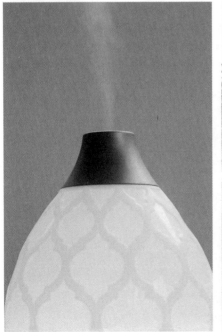

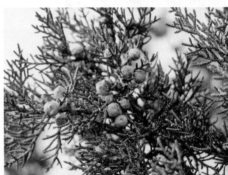

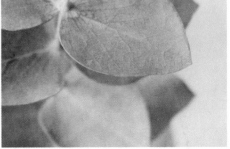

Chronic Low Immunity

If you seem to catch every cold that comes your way, it's best to focus on boosting your immune function for long-term support. Teachers are often prone to low immunity as stress can be high and they are sur-rounded by an influx of bacteria and viruses. The elderly are another susceptible group. A typical cold can quickly turn into pneumonia if not treated and monitored diligently. In general, I recommend using immunity tonics every fall, before cooler tempera-tures result in closed windows and doors, decreas-ing fresh air accessibility.

Immune-Defense Mushroom Capsules

½ ounce reishi powder
½ ounce lion's mane powder
½ ounce maitake powder
½ ounce shiitake powder

Mix the powdered herbs in a bowl and fill 200 empty capsules. Take 2 once or twice a day for 3 to 4 weeks.

Guard's-Up Tincture

3 teaspoons echinacea root
an additional 2 teaspoons echinacea root
2 ounces vodka

Put the 3 teaspoons of echinacea root in a 2-ounce jar and add vodka to fill. Close tightly and shake well. Keep in a pantry or cupboard for 3 weeks, shaking every day. Strain and add another teaspoon of echinacea root to the tincture. Again, close tightly and shake well. Keep in a pantry or cupboard for another 3 weeks. Strain and repeat one last time. You have now created a super-charged echinacea tincture. When you are heading into treacherous waters—planes or buses or trains, highly populated places, hospitals, schools, and the like—take 5 drops. At the first sign of a cold, take 5 drops 3 times a day for 2 days.

Build-My-Defense Tea

1 ounce astragalus root

1 ounce ashwagandha root

1 ounce reishi mushroom

½ ounce angelica root

½ ounce licorice root

Mix the herbs in a bowl and store in a glass jar. Steep 4 to 5 tablespoons in a quart of water. Drink 3 cups a day for 3 to 4 weeks.

Immune-Defense Balm

2 tablespoons rosemary leaf

1 tablespoon lavender flower

1 tablespoon lemon balm leaf

¾ cup olive oil

½ ounce beeswax

40–60 drops essential oil of your choice: frankincense, lavender, myrtle, clove, citrus, sandalwood, vetiver, or chamomile

Put the herbs in a glass baking dish and cover with olive oil to a depth of 1 or 2 inches. Bake at 170 degrees F for 4 hours. Allow to cool and then strain. Pour the oil into a saucepan and add the beeswax. Gently heat until the beeswax is melted. Add essential oils of your choice to reach your scent preference. Apply to the neck and chest each morning before leaving the house.

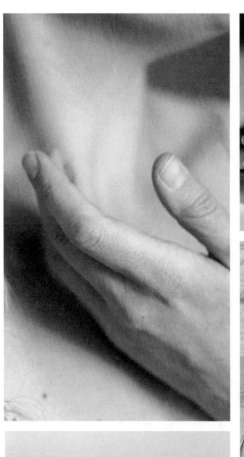

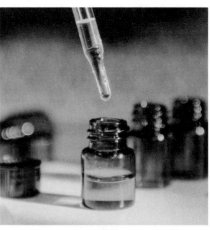

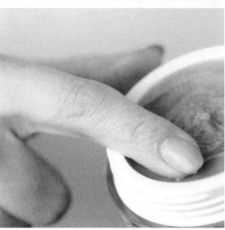

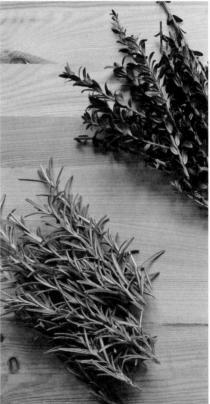

Circulation

Circulation comprises all of the pathways of the blood. It is directed by the pumping of the heart, which generates force to push the blood throughout the body. Sometimes smaller vessels become compromised, collapse, or are compressed by surrounding tissues. Other times if the heart isn't pumping with the same force it once was, it can be harder to get the blood to distal locations. This can lead to what is called poor circulation. The result is cold hands and feet, varicose veins, fatigue, and numbness and tingling.

Healthy-Circulation Tonic Tea

Taking a circulation tonic can support the system by toning the vessels and opening channels that may be compromised.

1 ounce hawthorn berry

1 ounce bilberry fruit

½ ounce hawthorn leaf and flower

½ ounce ginkgo leaf

½ ounce horse chestnut

½ ounce ginger root

Mix the herbs in a bowl and store in a glass jar. Use 4 to 5 table-spoons to make 1-quart batches. Drink 1 to 3 cups per day for 8 to 12 weeks if desiring a tonic effect. Alternatively, you can drink 1 cup as desired for intermittent circulation support.

Coughs

Coughs are never simple. Understanding what is driving them helps to pinpoint the best herbs to relieve them. I believe a two- or three-pronged approach is best with coughs—tea and tincture as well as something topical—to kick them out of the respiratory system. For babies and children, please see the special section on page 186.

Dry-Cough Tea

1 ounce mullein leaf

1 ounce marshmallow root

1 ounce wild cherry bark

½ ounce violet leaf

½ ounce licorice root

Mix the herbs in a bowl and store in a glass jar. Steep 4 to 5 tablespoons in a quart of water. Drink 3 cups a day for 3 to 4 weeks.

Wet-Cough Tea

1 ounce elecampane root

1 ounce rosemary leaf

1 ounce osha root

½ ounce sage root

½ ounce licorice root

Mix the herbs in a bowl and store in a glass jar. Steep 4 to 5 tablespoons in a quart of water. Drink 3 cups a day for 3 to 4 weeks.

Dry-Cough Tincture

1 teaspoon mullein leaf

1 teaspoon marshmallow root

1 teaspoon wild cherry bark

½ teaspoon violet leaf

½ teaspoon licorice root

2 ounces vodka or apple cider vinegar

Put the herbs in a 2-ounce jar and add vodka or apple cider vinegar to fill. Close tightly and shake well. Keep in a pantry or cupboard for 3 weeks, shaking every day. Strain and transfer to a 2-ounce dropper bottle. Take 2 dropperfuls 4 times daily when cough is present.

Wet-Cough Tincture

Best to have this formulated at your local herb shop for you.

20 milliliters usnea tincture

20 milliliters osha root tincture

10 milliliters rosemary leaf tincture

5 milliliters marshmallow root tincture

5 milliliters elecampane root tincture

Mix the tinctures in a 2-ounce dropper bottle. Take 2 dropperfuls 4 times daily when cough is present.

Expectorant Tea

When you've got phlegm and it just isn't moving, try this tea. Be sure to drink it hot to allow the volatile oils to roll off the steam as you drink.

1 ounce elderberry

1 ounce spearmint leaf

½ ounce elderflower

½ ounce nettle leaf

½ ounce hyssop leaf and flower

½ ounce black cohosh root

Mix the herbs in a bowl and store in a glass jar. Steep 4 to 5 tablespoons in a quart of water. Drink 3 cups a day as long as needed.

Cough-Quell Syrup

1 ounce wild cherry bark

1 ounce marshmallow root

1 ounce hyssop leaf

½ ounce mullein leaf

½ ounce yerba santa leaf

8 cups water

3 cups cane sugar or honey

¼ cup apple cider vinegar

Put the herbs in a saucepan with the water. Bring to a boil and reduce by half on a medium-low heat. Strain out the herbs and put the brew back into the pan. Add sugar or honey and gently heat to mix if necessary, stirring continuously. Turn off the heat, add the apple cider vinegar, and allow to cool. Then transfer to your container of choice and store in the refrigerator. Take 1 teaspoon as needed.

The steamy shower remedy

Taking a steamy shower usually helps relieve symptoms when the respiratory system is compromised. Pounding (gently) on your chest can aid circulation and break up phlegm. Add a few drops of eucalyptus or rosemary essential oils to your shower for a therapeutic effect.

Ditch-the-Cough Essential Oil Blend

This oil blend can help you sleep when coughing is keeping you awake through the night.

4 drops ravensara essential oil

2 drops eucalyptus radiata essential oil

2 drops lavender essential oil

2 drops valerian essential oil

1 drop pine essential oil

1 ounce apricot oil

Blend the oils in a 1-ounce bottle and gently shake. Apply a couple of drops to the upper back and top of the chest before bed.

Herbal Cough Drops

You will need a cough drop mold for this.

1 ounce horehound leaf

1 ounce marshmallow root

1 ounce mullein leaf

½ ounce licorice root

½ ounce cinnamon chips

¾ cup honey

Mix the herbs in a bowl and store in a glass jar. Add 4 tablespoons to a pint of hot water, close, and let steep overnight. Strain in the morning and put the infusion in a saucepan. Turn the heat on low and add honey. Bring to a boil until the liquid reaches 300 degrees F, and then pour into your mold. Allow to cool and wrap each drop in waxed paper. Store in a jar in the refrigerator. Allow to dissolve in mouth as needed.

Travel Cough Lozenges

Sitting on a plane with a cough is the worst. Having these lozenges to soothe the cough and boost your immune defenses will make you, and your neighbor, much happier.

½ tablespoon horehound leaf

½ tablespoon sage leaf

½ tablespoon wild cherry bark

1 teaspoon ashwagandha root

1 teaspoon chamomile flower

¾ cup boiling water

¾ cup honey

5–10 drops sweet orange essential oil

slippery elm bark powder

Steep the herbs in the boiling water for 1 hour and then strain and pour into a small saucepan. Add the honey and heat over medium heat just until the mixture begins to boil. Using a candy thermometer, determine when the temperature reaches 300 degrees F and then turn off the heat. Let the mixture cool for 5 to 10 minutes, until it starts to get syrupy. Add the essential oil. Drop by small spoonfuls onto parchment paper and let cool. Dust with slippery elm bark powder and once they are completely cooled, store in a glass jar. Melt in mouth as needed.

Cuts & Scrapes

It's better not to ignore even tiny cuts. If a cut or scrape is red, streaking, swollen, tender, pus producing, or throbbing, it is stressing your immune system and needs treatment.

Herbal Wound Spray

Using a spray on a wound to clean it before applying a salve can greatly reduce the risk of infection.

1 teaspoon calendula flower

1 teaspoon sage leaf

1 teaspoon yarrow leaf and flower

1 teaspoon goldenseal root

1 teaspoon myrrh resin

6 ounces hot water

½ ounce aloe vera juice

½ ounce witch hazel extract

sage essential oil

lavender essential oil

Steep the herbs in the hot water for 2 hours. Strain and put 1 ounce of the infusion in a 2-ounce spray bottle. Add the aloe vera juice, witch hazel extract, and essential oils. Gently shake to combine everything. Spray this onto a wound and dab with a cotton pad.

Antibacterial Salve

Having a salve to apply topically can serve a multitude of purposes. You can use it for cuts and scrapes to keep the area sealed off from infection, and you can also use it as lip balm or lip protector from strong weather elements.

1 tablespoon calendula flower

1 tablespoon goldenseal root

½ tablespoon comfrey leaf

½ tablespoon lemon balm leaf

½ tablespoon chickweed leaf

½ tablespoon lavender flower

¾ cup olive oil

½ ounce beeswax

40 drops lemon essential oil

20 drops thyme essential oil

Put the herbs in a glass baking dish and cover with olive oil to a depth of 1 or 2 inches. Bake at 170 degrees F for 4 hours. Allow to cool and then strain. Pour the oil into a saucepan and add the beeswax. Gently heat until the beeswax is melted. Pour into your container of choice and add essential oils. Slather it on cuts and scrapes as needed.

Diarrhea

Diarrhea can come on from many causes. It can be acute from a bacterial or viral infection or from spoiled food or water. It can also take a chronic form caused by stress, a low-grade infection, or improper digestive flora. One thing to always keep in mind when diarrhea strikes is the need to stay hydrated. Diarrhea is extremely dehydrating, as it pulls enormous amounts of water from the body.

Diarrhea-Stop Capsules

I typically recommend capsules for diarrhea because the medicine passes directly through the digestive system. That being said, this can easily be converted to drops if you prefer or are worried about too much elimination occurring for the medicine to get effectively broken down and utilized.

½ ounce plantain leaf powder

½ ounce sage leaf powder

¼ ounce goldenseal root powder

¼ ounce raspberry leaf powder

¼ ounce slippery elm bark powder

¼ ounce echinacea root powder

Mix the powdered herbs in a bowl and fill 200 empty capsules. Take 2 capsules every 2 to 3 hours until symptoms subside.

Acute-Diarrhea Tincture

1 teaspoon Oregon grape root

1 teaspoon goldenseal root

1 teaspoon licorice root

2 teaspoons raspberry leaf

2 ounces vodka or apple cider vinegar

Put the herbs in a 2-ounce jar and add vodka or apple cider vinegar to fill. Close tightly and shake well. Keep in a pantry or cupboard for 3 weeks, shaking every day. Strain and transfer to a 2-ounce dropper bottle. Take 2 dropperfuls 3 times a day for 3 to 5 days when diarrhea strikes. Continue taking 1 day past the resolution of symptoms.

Intestine-Calming Essential Oil Blend

This blend has proven to calm the overactivity of the lower intestines.

20 drops frankincense essential oil

20 drops chamomile essential oil

10 drops fennel essential oil

5 drops lavender essential oil

4 ounces hemp oil

Blend all ingredients in a 4-ounce bottle. Rub 1 to 2 teaspoons into the skin of the abdomen when needed.

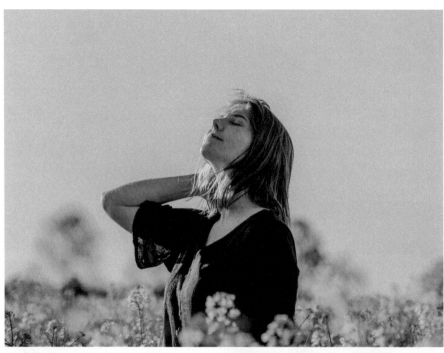

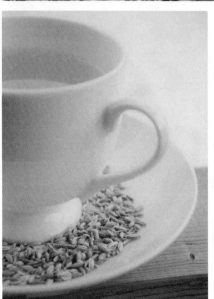

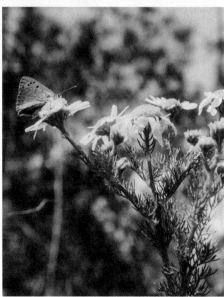

Earaches

The typical earache is usually caused by a bacterial infection, but it can also be viral. Calming inflammation and ridding the ear of infection are the keys to treatment. Massaging the ear also helps to drain fluid if pressure is a problem. Remember, the eardrum or tympanic membrane is a protective wall. Don't stick Q-tips or anything similar into the ear, as rupture is common. Although it can heal, the tympanic membrane is an important barrier between the inside and outside structures of the ear. If you are suffering from an earache and find a bit of blood on your pillow upon waking, it is likely the tympanic membrane has ruptured, and it is advisable to see a practitioner.

Ear Infection Calming Tincture

2 teaspoons echinacea root

1 teaspoon chamomile flower

½ teaspoon red root

½ teaspoon licorice root

2 ounces vodka or apple cider vinegar

Put the herbs in a 2-ounce jar and add vodka or apple cider vinegar to fill. Close tightly and shake well. Keep in a pantry or cupboard for 3 weeks, shaking every day. Strain and transfer to a 2-ounce dropper bottle. Take 1 or 2 dropperfuls 3 times a day as needed.

Earache-Soothing Tea

1 ounce elderberry

1 ounce echinacea root

1 ounce lemon balm leaf

½ ounce chamomile flower

½ ounce licorice root

Mix the herbs in a bowl and store in a glass jar. Make tea by the cup. Steep 1 or 2 teaspoons in 10 ounces of hot water, covered, for 10 minutes. Drink as needed.

Rose-Petal Earache Infusion

2 teaspoons dried rose petals

8 ounces of water

Heat the water to boiling and steep the petals for 20 minutes. Trickle the warm infusion into the ear and allow it to rest there for a few minutes.

Earache Pain Relief Oil

1 ounce arnica-infused oil

1 ounce poplar-infused oil

Mix the oils together. Apply a little bit behind and below the ear and massage all around the exterior surface of the ear.

Onion Poultice for Earache

This is an old recipe I've used a lot.

1 yellow onion

1 tablespoon olive oil

flour of your choice

Dice the onion and sauté in olive oil until translucent. Pull from the heat and add just enough flour to make a thick paste. Find an old sock that has lost its mate and stuff it with the paste. Lay this warm sock over the ear or behind the ear for pain and congestion relief.

Mullein-Garlic Oil for Earache

Throughout summer, the herb mullein grows big, beautiful stalks packed with delicate yellow flowers. These flowers have long been used to soothe ear problems. When combined with garlic, you have an antibacterial force to be reckoned with. You only get the fresh flowers in summer, so you have to make your year's supply all at once.

fresh mullein flowers

fresh garlic cloves

olive oil

Fill a 4-ounce jar with mullein flowers and add olive oil to the top. Fill another 4-ounce jar with garlic cloves and add olive oil to the top. Close the jars and set out in the sun for 4 weeks, shaking daily. Every couple of days, take the lids off for a few hours to allow for water evaporation. You'll need steady temperatures to make this solar infusion, 80 degrees F or higher. After both the oils are done, strain them. Mix 1 ounce of the mullein flower oil with 1/2 ounce of the garlic oil. To use, warm up slightly in the palms of your hand, drop 1 or 2 drops directly into the ear, and massage the ear gently. I gently pull up, down, and back on the ear lobe and then massage behind the ear. Can be done 3 times a day.

Fevers

By design, fevers are our body's way of making our insides inhospitable to foreign invaders. Sometimes our body struggles to mount a fever, allowing illness to bloom. Other times fevers flare too high for too long, which can lead to a debilitated state. Encouraging them to follow their natural course can be hard, particularly when the fever compromises sleep or comfort. While over-the-counter fever reducers aid our comfort level, they often create a rebound effect, which can lead to a higher fever and prolonged illness. Trust your body, find the balance you are comfortable with, and consider these recipes for support. For babies and children, please see the special section on page 190.

Fever-Breaking Yarrow Tea

1 teaspoon yarrow flower

Steep in 10 ounces of hot water, covered, for 10 minutes. Drink hot every few hours until fever breaks. Stop if excessive sweating is occurring so as not to reach exhaustion.

Fever-Reducer Capsules

½ ounce white willow bark
½ ounce elderflower
½ ounce holy basil leaf
½ ounce chamomile flower

Mix the powdered herbs in a bowl and fill 200 empty capsules. Take 2 every 4 hours.

Fever-Tamer Tea

This tea helps when a fever is running too high for too long.

¾ ounce boneset leaf

½ ounce sage leaf

½ ounce white willow bark

½ ounce fenugreek seeds

½ ounce catnip leaf

¼ ounce licorice root

Mix the herbs in a bowl and store in a glass jar. Make tea by the cup. Steep 1 or 2 teaspoons in 10 ounces of hot water, covered, for 10 minutes. Drink hot every few hours until the fever breaks.

Fever-Cooling Compress

8 ounces cold water

30 drops rosemary essential oil

10 drops peppermint essential oil

Add the essential oils to the water and stir. Quickly soak a cotton cloth in water, wring it out, and apply it to the forehead or the nape of the neck. Refresh every 30 minutes, stirring the water each time before immersing the cloth.

A trick
to encourage a fever

Try drinking hot ginger or elderflower tea while taking a hot bath to encourage a fever and light perspiration.

Head Colds

A simple head cold can be combated with so many herbal and nature-cure options that there is no need to let it run its course without helping your body fight it. The congestion, headache, runny nose, sore throat, and cough that come along with it can be diminished with just a cup of tea or a few doses of tincture throughout. Be sure to check out individual sections on those things for targeted recipes. Following are great remedies to have in your medicine chest so when the sneezing and runny nose begin, you are prepared for battle. For babies and children, please see the special section on page 192.

Cold-Care Capsules

This general blend is to target basic cold symptoms of runny nose, congestion, and respiratory complaints.

½ ounce myrrh powder

½ ounce yarrow leaf and flower powder

¼ ounce usnea lichen powder

¼ ounce lion's mane mushroom powder

¼ ounce horehound leaf powder

¼ ounce ginger root powder

Mix the powdered herbs in a bowl and fill 200 empty capsules. Take 2 capsules 4 times a day as needed.

Breathe-Easier Tea

This blend includes herbs with a high volatile oil content that work great to open up the nasal passageways. Be sure to steep the blend covered, because otherwise the oils can evaporate with the steam. Best to drink this tea hot, as it'll help break up the phlegm.

1 ounce spearmint leaf

1 ounce peppermint leaf

½ ounce boneset leaf

½ ounce yarrow leaf and flower

½ ounce elderflower

½ ounce rosehips

Mix the herbs in a bowl and store in a glass jar. Make tea by the cup. Steep 1 or 2 teaspoons in 10 ounces of hot water, covered, for 10 minutes.

Neti pots for respiratory support

I am a big proponent of neti pots and encourage their regular use, particularly during allergy and cold seasons. The practice of washing out the nose and sinus cavities aids in keeping the system free of irritating particles and excessive mucus. I for one cannot sleep without breathing through my nose, and when a cold has completely blocked that ability, a neti pot can be a life saver.

Stop-the-Drip Tincture

When your nose is runny and you are completely blocked, it's torture. When I lean over the sink to do the dishes and my nose drips out of control, I've reached my limit with head cold symptoms. Try this formula to dry up the drip and open up the nasal passageways.

2 teaspoons myrrh resin

1 teaspoon chaga mushroom powder

½ teaspoon goldenseal root

½ teaspoon poke root

2 ounces vodka

Put the herbs in a 2-ounce jar and add vodka to fill. Close tightly and shake well. Keep in a pantry or cupboard for 3 weeks, shaking every day. Strain and transfer to a 2-ounce dropper bottle. Take 1 to 2 dropperfuls 3 times a day until symptoms subside.

Congestion-Breakup Capsules

1 ounce myrrh powder

¼ ounce anise seed powder

½ ounce holy basil leaf powder

¼ ounce Oregon grape root powder

⅛ ounce cayenne powder

Use gloves due to cayenne power. Mix the powdered herbs in a bowl and fill 200 empty capsules. Take 2 capsules every 3 hours as needed.

Decongesting Herbal Steam

This is a good treatment before work or bed to open up the upper respiratory system. If you have access to fresh herbs, use them as the volatile oils are more abundant. You can also combine fresh and dried herbs as needed, or use just the dried herbs if that is what is available to you.

1 ½ ounces lemon peel

1 ounce thyme leaf

½ ounce rosemary leaf

½ ounce peppermint leaf

½ ounce eucalyptus leaf

Combine the herbs and store in a glass jar. When needed, bring 8 to 12 cups of water to a boil in a large stockpot. Turn off the heat and add a handful or two of the herbal blend. Close the lid and let steep for 5 minutes. Take the lid off to allow the steam to roll off a bit to ensure you don't burn your face. Get a bath towel and cover your head and shoulders from behind. Lean over the pot until you feel the steam and can breathe in the scent. Stay as long as comfortable—feel free to do little stints then take a break. Cover the pot in between to preserve the heat and volatile oils in the steam.

Decongesting Vapor Balm

2 tablespoons eucalyptus leaf

1 tablespoon thyme leaf

1 tablespoon rosemary leaf

¾ cup olive oil

½ ounce beeswax

pine and fir essential oils

Put the herbs in a glass baking dish and cover with olive oil to a depth of 1 or 2 inches. Bake at 170 degrees F for 4 hours. Allow to cool and then strain. Pour the oil into a saucepan and add the beeswax. Gently heat until the beeswax is melted. Pour into your container of choice and add the essential oils. Rub a bit of balm onto the neck, under the nose, and onto the chest, and inhale. Reapply as needed.

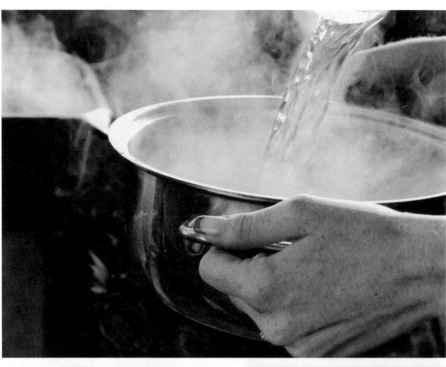

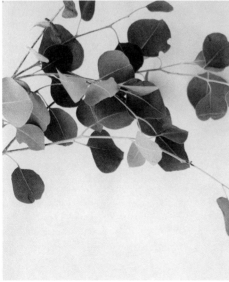

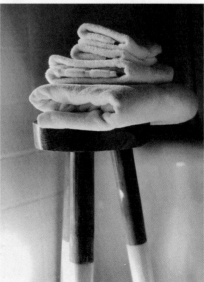

Immune Boost

These recipes are preventive and will help you stay healthy during the onslaught of wintertime colds and flus. They are not recommended for acute situations. If you are the type of person who catches every cold that comes through, consider the recipes in the section "Chronic Low Immunity."

Immune-Boost Tea

Drink this from time to time throughout the year to keep the immune system sharp and ready.

1 ounce astragalus root

1 ounce holy basil leaf

¾ ounce elderberry

½ ounce olive leaf

½ ounce ginkgo leaf

¼ ounce ginger root

Mix the herbs in a bowl and store in a glass jar. Steep 4 or 5 tablespoons in a quart of hot water overnight. Strain and drink 3 cups a day, either occasionally or for 1 to 2 weeks at a time to support the immune system.

Bug-Defense Capsules

½ ounce olive leaf powder

½ ounce eleuthero root powder

¼ ounce astragalus root powder

¼ ounce elecampane root powder

¼ ounce mullein leaf powder

⅛ ounce ginger root powder

⅛ ounce cinnamon bark powder

Mix the powdered herbs in a bowl and fill 200 empty capsules. Take 2 twice per day for 2 to 3 days as needed.

Fire Cider

Rosemary Gladstar first concocted fire cider, a spicy hot, deliciously sweet vinegar tonic, in the kitchen at the California School of Herbal Studies in the early 1980s. Fire cider has been at the center of a trademark controversy, but as Gladstar states on her website Freefirecider.com, fire cider is for everyone to use. Here is one recipe, but there are countless others out there. Get creative and customize your own blend. Use it to boost your immune system and combat colds and flus, particularly bacterial types. A shot a day keeps the doctor away.

½ cup fresh grated ginger root

½ cup fresh grated horseradish root

1 onion, chopped

10 cloves garlic, crushed

zest and juice from 1 lemon

2 whole astragalus roots

2 sprigs fresh or dried rosemary leaf

1 tablespoon turmeric powder

¼ teaspoon cayenne powder

organic apple cider vinegar

¼ to ⅓ cup raw local honey (optional)

Place the herbs in a quart jar and cover with apple cider vinegar, leaving 1 inch of headroom at the top. Insert a piece of parchment paper under the lid to keep the vinegar from touching the metal. Shake well and store in a cool, dark place for 6 to 8 weeks, shaking gently daily. Use cheesecloth to strain out the pulp, pouring the vinegar into a clean jar. Be sure to squeeze as much of the liquid from the pulp as you can; you may want to wear gloves as it can cause skin irritation. If you want to add honey, do it now. Heating the mixture isn't a great idea as it can destroy the probiotic healing property of vinegar, but you can gently heat the honey on low if needed and then add it to the vinegar.

Germ-Blaster Potpourri

Having these scented herbs in the open airways of your home can not only promote energy, relaxation, or focus but also combat winter colds and flus. Choose a pretty bowl and set it out for display—the volatile oils will waft into the air, but you can also rub some between your hands before taking a nice big inhalation. Alternatively, you can make simmering potpourri by simply adding the ingredients to a simmer pot on the stove.

2 handfuls of each of the following: lavender, cedar, bitter
orange peel, lemon balm, hibiscus, juniper berries, star anise,
and rose petals

1–2 tablespoons orris root powder

10 drops spruce essential oil

5 drops clove essential oil

5 drops ginger essential oil

5 drops lemon essential oil

Mix the herbs in a bowl with the orris root powder and essential oils. Put into an airtight container for 1 to 2 weeks to allow to set, and then it's ready to go!

Immune-System-Up Travel Drops

Before I get on a plane I take a dropperful of this blend to tell my immune system to be on the alert. You can also take this a couple of days before a trip, especially when you are traveling long distances and sleep will be compromised.

2 teaspoons reishi mushroom

1 teaspoon ashwagandha root

1 teaspoon nettle leaf

½ teaspoon spirulina

½ teaspoon rosehips

2 ounces vodka

Put the herbs in a 2-ounce jar and add vodka to fill. Close tightly and shake well. Keep in a pantry or cupboard for 3 weeks, shaking every day. Strain and transfer to a 2-ounce dropper bottle. Take 1 dropperful right before plane, train, or bus travel.

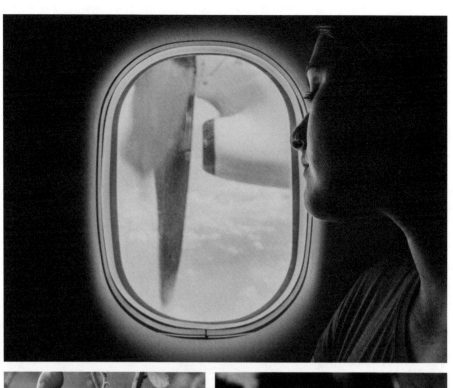

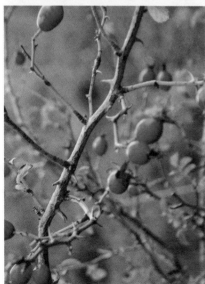

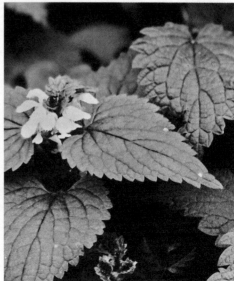

Influenza, a.k.a. the Flu

Flus can be bacterial or viral, but both typically take us out of the daily living game. Body aches, headache, vomiting, diarrhea, and overall malaise are what most people report. I'm always curious when a flu rages through our household. While it's obvious that we've all contracted the same illness, it tends to present itself slightly differently in each of my family members. For me, vomiting is inevitable; my husband gets excruciating back and hip pain; my son aches all over and can never get comfortable; and my daughter seems to take it in stride, setting up camp in bed but able to enjoy the extra attention and cuddles. Luckily, and knock on wood, my husband and I tag team each other when the flu shows up, taking just one of us down at a time. For treating the flu, the keys are support, finding comfort, hydration, and rest.

Flu-Fighter Tea

Sipping this tea throughout the day keeps hydration up and provides the body with mini shots of herbal fighting power against the invasion.

1 ounce chamomile flower

1 ounce rosehips

1 ounce lemon balm leaf

½ ounce boneset leaf

½ ounce yarrow flower

Mix the herbs in a bowl and store in a glass jar. Make tea by the cup. Steep 1 or 2 teaspoons in 10 ounces of hot water, covered, for 10 minutes. Sip throughout the day.

Flu-Fighter Capsules

½ ounce boneset leaf powder

½ ounce elderflower powder

½ ounce activated charcoal

⅛ ounce echinacea root powder

⅛ ounce California poppy powder

⅛ ounce hops powder

⅛ ounce catnip leaf powder

Mix the powdered herbs in a bowl and fill 200 empty capsules. Take 2 capsules every 3 hours until symptoms subside.

Flu-Fighter Essential Oil Diffuser Blend

Flu comes on? Have the diffuser on 24/7.

5 milliliters lemon essential oil

3 milliliters lavender essential oil

2 milliliters rosemary essential oil

Blend in a 10-milliliter essential oil bottle. Drop 5 drops into the diffuser as needed.

Castor oil flu treatment

Apply a castor oil pack to the abdomen twice daily to stimulate immune system circulation and clear toxins from the body. This is relatively easy to do even when you are wiped out and creates a level of comfort that allows you to relax. Rub 2 tablespoons castor oil over the abdomen. Cover with a cotton towel and then a hot water bottle or heating pad. Relax for 30 to 45 minutes, or put on before bed and go to sleep.

Laryngitis

Laryngitis is an inflammation of the voice box that can cause hoarseness or complete loss of the voice. Treatments directly applied to the throat are important and are best coupled with internal treatment.

Laryngitis-Soothing Gargle

1 ounce barberry root

1 ounce echinacea root

1 ounce marshmallow root

½ ounce turmeric root

½ ounce goldenseal root

¼ cup apple cider vinegar

Mix the herbs together and store in a glass jar. Steep 4 table-spoons in a pint of hot water overnight. Strain and add the apple cider vinegar. Store in the refrigerator for up to 5 days. Gargle 1 or 2 ounces several times throughout the day as needed.

Laryngitis Lozenges

2 ounces horehound leaf

1 ounce slippery elm bark

1 ounce chamomile flower

1 ounce ginger root

¾ cup honey

Mix the herbs in a bowl and store in a glass jar. Steep 4 table-spoons in a pint of hot water overnight. Strain in the morning and put the infusion in a saucepan. Turn the heat on low and add the honey, heating until it reaches 300 degrees F. Then pour into a lozenge mold, allow to cool, and wrap each lozenge in waxed paper. Store in a jar in the refrigerator and melt one lozenge in the mouth as needed.

Voice-Restoring Tea

1 ounce thyme leaf

1 ounce marshmallow root

½ ounce mullein leaf

½ ounce coltsfoot leaf

½ ounce licorice root

½ ounce rose petals

Mix the herbs in a bowl and store in a glass jar. Make tea by the cup. Steep 1 or 2 teaspoons in 10 ounces of hot water, covered, for 10 minutes.

Diffuser Blend for Laryngitis

7 milliliters rosemary essential oil

2 milliliters peppermint essential oil

1 milliliter black pepper essential oil

Mix the oils in a 10-milliliter essential oil bottle. Drop 5 drops into your diffuser as needed.

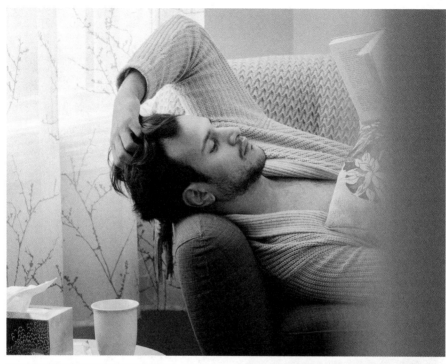

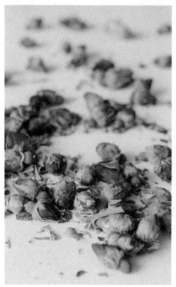

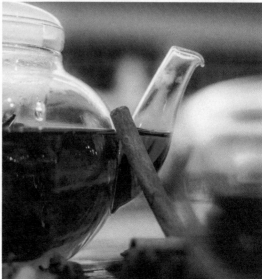

Pink Eye (Conjunctivitis)

Pink eye is a very common and very contagious infection. It presents as redness of the eye, often accompanied by itching and weepiness. It can be caused by viruses, bacteria, irritations, or allergies. The formulas included here target bacterial conjunctivitis but will help relieve eye irritations of any kind. Keep the kiddos home from school when they have pink eye to prevent contaminating others. Frequent hand washing is important, along with disinfecting things like keyboards, remote controls, and toys.

Pink-Eye Wash

1 ounce calendula flower
1 ounce Oregon grape root
1 ounce myrrh resin
½ ounce chamomile flower
½ ounce chickweed leaf

Mix the herbs in a bowl and store in a glass jar until needed. Steep 5 tablespoons in a pint of hot water for 2 hours or overnight. Strain and keep in the refrigerator for up to 4 days. Saturate a cotton ball for each eye and use it to drench the eye above, below, and inside. Do not reuse cotton balls or use the same one for both eyes. Dab with a hand towel afterward. Do this 4 to 6 times a day during active infection.

Pink-Eye Tincture

Take this tincture at the same time to fight the infection internally.

1 teaspoon echinacea root
1 teaspoon licorice root
½ teaspoon dandelion root
½ teaspoon blackberry leaf
½ teaspoon Oregon grape root
½ teaspoon calendula flower
2 ounces vodka or apple cider vinegar

Put the herbs in a 2-ounce jar and add vodka or apple cider vinegar to fill. Close tightly and shake well. Keep in a pantry or cupboard for 3 weeks, shaking every day. Strain and transfer to a 2-ounce dropper bottle. Take 2 dropperfuls 3 times a day during acute infection.

Sinusitis

A respiratory infection often results in a sinus infection, or for some, sinus infections just develop all
on their own. I've repeatedly discovered with my
chronic sinusitis patients that diet clearly plays
a role, and there is often a direct correlation with
sugar, gluten, and dairy intake. Committing to an
anti-inflammatory diet has greatly reduced the frequency and severity of chronic or repeated sinus
infections for most of my patients. Being diligent
with self-care once a sinus infection is suspected
can greatly reduce symptoms and discomfort.

Sinusitis-Relief Infusion

The age-old tradition of washing out the nasal passageways helps to clear them of sinusitis-causing germs. It can also increase breathing capacity and soothe the membranes of the upper respiratory tract. Several of my patients who suffered tremendously from chronic sinus infections have found relief with the use of a neti pot in the treatment plan. Even if you are completely blocked, using a neti pot can eventually break through the wall of mucus and provide sweet relief. Try using just salt first, 1 teaspoon to 16 ounces of lukewarm water. Then try this infusion.

1 tablespoon marshmallow root
1 tablespoon goldenseal root

Steep the herbs in 8 ounces of room temperature water for 2 hours or overnight. Strain and save the herbs for reuse. For an active sinus infection, blend 1 teaspoon salt, 2 ounces of the infusion, and 12 ounces of lukewarm water and run it through the sinuses. If you suspect mold is an issue, add 1 dropperful of black walnut hull tincture to 16 ounces of lukewarm water.

Sinus-Relief Capsules

½ ounce hyssop leaf powder
½ ounce myrrh resin powder
½ ounce nettle leaf powder
¼ ounce fennel seed powder
⅛ ounce horseradish powder

Mix the powdered herbs in a bowl and fill 200 empty capsules. Take 2 capsules 3 times a day until symptoms subside.

Sinus-Relief Tea

1¼ ounces orange peel

1 ounce rosehips

½ ounce hyssop leaf

½ ounce mullein leaf

½ ounce thyme leaf

¼ ounce licorice root

Mix the herbs in a bowl and store in a glass jar. Make tea by the cup. Steep 1 or 2 teaspoons in 10 ounces of hot water, covered, for 10 minutes. Sip throughout the day.

Sinus Balm

2 tablespoons rosemary leaf

2 tablespoons elderflower

1 tablespoon white willow bark

1 tablespoon plantain leaf

¾ cup olive oil

½ ounce beeswax

40 drops pine essential oil

15 drops geranium essential oil

5 drops benzoin essential oil

Put the herbs in a glass baking dish and cover with olive oil to a depth of 1 or 2 inches. Bake at 170 degrees F for 4 hours. Allow to cool and then strain. Pour the oil into a saucepan and add the beeswax. Gently heat until the beeswax is melted. Pour into your container of choice and add essential oils. Rub this on your forehead and nose for temporary relief of sinus pain and pressure.

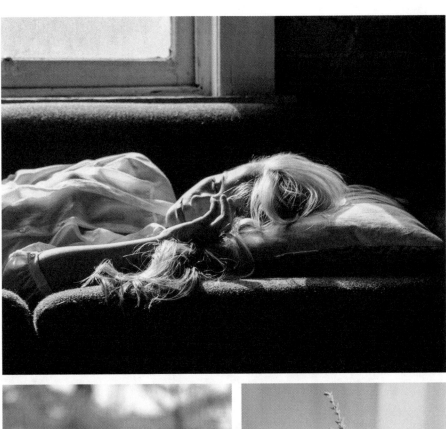

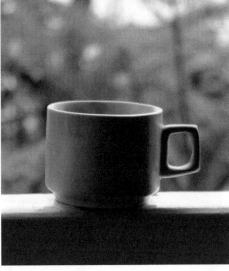

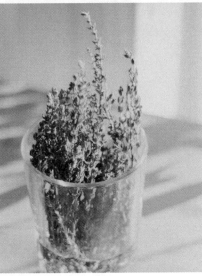

Sore Throat

My red flag that illness is hovering is a sore throat. Having suffered from chronic strep throat as a child, I know this is my susceptible point—when I feel that all-too-familiar sensation, I get on it. Most sore throats that are part of a cold are caused by viral infections, while strep throat is bacterial. Sore throats can also be caused by allergies, air contaminants, digestive issues, and smoking. For babies and children, please see the special section on page 194.

Sore-Throat Spray

A topical blast directly onto the tissues can help ease the pain and fight the infection.

2 teaspoons prickly ash bark

1 teaspoon sage leaf

1 teaspoon echinacea root

½ teaspoon myrrh resin

1 ounce apple cider vinegar

1 ounce vegetable glycerin

Put the herbs in a 2-ounce jar and add apple cider vinegar and glycerin to fill. Close tightly and shake well. Keep in a pantry or cupboard for 3 weeks, shaking every day. Strain and transfer to a 2-ounce spray bottle. Spray 1 or 2 times into the mouth and toward the throat as needed.

Throat-Soothing Tea

2 ounces sage leaf

1 ounce mullein leaf

½ ounce slippery elm bark

½ ounce licorice root

⅛ ounce whole cloves

Mix the herbs in a bowl and store in a glass jar. Make tea by the cup. Steep 1 or 2 teaspoons in 10 ounces of hot water, covered, for 10 minutes. Sip as needed throughout the day.

Throat-Soothing Tincture

2 teaspoons sage leaf

1 teaspoon echinacea root

1 teaspoon hyssop leaf

½ teaspoon elderberry

½ teaspoon red root

2 ounces vodka or apple cider vinegar

Put the herbs in a 2-ounce jar and add vodka or apple cider vinegar to fill. Close tightly and shake well. Keep in a pantry or cupboard for 3 weeks, shaking every day. Strain and transfer to a 2-ounce dropper bottle. Take 1 or 2 dropperfuls 3 times a day.

Sore-Throat Lozenges

2 ounces rosehips

1 ounce slippery elm bark

1 ounce marshmallow root

1 ounce prickly ash bark

¾ cup honey

80–100 drops orange essential oil

Mix the herbs in a bowl and store in a glass jar. Steep 5 tablespoons in a pint of hot water overnight. Strain in the morning and put the infusion in a saucepan. Turn the heat on low and add the honey, heating until it reaches 300 degrees F. Allow to cool slightly and add the essential oil. Then pour into a lozenge mold, allow to cool, and wrap each lozenge in waxed paper. Store in a jar in the refrigerator and melt one lozenge in the mouth as needed.

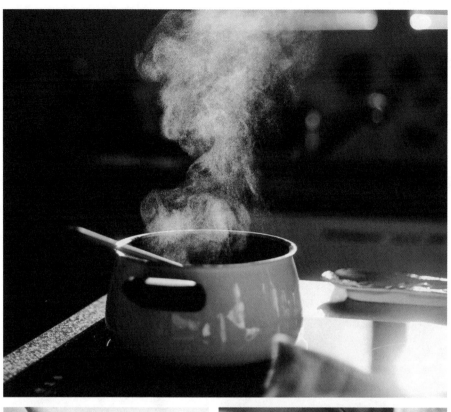

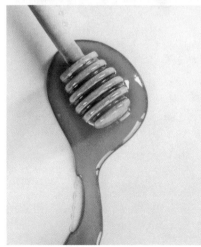

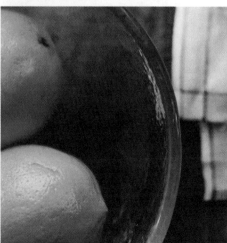

Staph Infections

Staph infections are bacterial and typically reside on the skin, but internal staph infections such as food poisoning and toxic shock syndrome are also possible. Considered highly contagious, staph often presents on the skin in the form of a boil, a furuncle, an abscess, or a collection of pus. It can also present with a crust that looks like dried honey, typical of impetigo. Keep the area clean and disinfected to resolve the infection. Honey has been used as an effective healing agent for staph infections for centuries.

Staph-Fighting Spray

Use this spray to fight infection and keep the area clean.

½ ounce lavender flower

½ ounce calendula flower

½ ounce yarrow flower

½ ounce goldenseal root

12 ounces distilled water

3 ounces apple cider vinegar

1 ounce vodka

Put the herbs in a pint jar and add the distilled water, apple cider vinegar, and vodka. Close tightly and shake well. Keep in a pantry or cupboard for 3 weeks, shaking every day. Strain and transfer to a 2-ounce spray bottle. Spray onto the affected area 4 times a day, allowing it to dry. Alternatively, you can spray a cotton pad and affix it to the area with gauze, changing the dressing 3 times a day.

Staph-Fighting Tincture

Best to support the body from the inside out when dealing with staph infections.

2 teaspoons echinacea root

1 teaspoon Oregon grape root

1 teaspoon usnea, cut up finely

1 teaspoon calendula flower

2 ounces vodka or apple cider vinegar

Put the herbs in a 2-ounce jar and add vodka or apple cider vinegar to fill. Close tightly and shake well. Keep in a pantry or cupboard for 3 weeks, shaking every day. Strain and transfer to a 2-ounce dropper bottle. Take 1 or 2 dropperfuls 3 times a day.

Strep Throat

See also "Sore Throat." The following recipes are specific to strep throat infections.

Strep-Relief Tea

1 ounce echinacea root

1 ounce orange peel

½ ounce osha root

½ ounce hyssop leaf

½ ounce sage leaf

½ ounce wild cherry bark

Mix the herbs in a bowl and store in a glass jar. Make tea by the cup. Steep 1 or 2 teaspoons in 10 ounces of hot water, covered, for 10 minutes. Drink 3 cups a day, sweetening with honey to taste.

Strep-Fighting Tincture

2 teaspoons echinacea root

1 teaspoon wireweed leaf

1 teaspoon lomatium root

1 teaspoon sage leaf

2 ounces vodka or apple cider vinegar

Put the herbs in a 2-ounce jar and add vodka or apple cider vinegar to fill. Close tightly and shake well. Keep in a pantry or cupboard for 3 weeks, shaking every day. Strain and transfer to a 2-ounce dropper bottle. Take 2 dropperfuls, holding it in the mouth for 30 seconds and then allowing it to slowly slide into the throat before swallowing.

Swollen Glands

When the glands in your neck and throat area are swollen, your body is trying to tell you something. Respond with these recipes to support the lymphatic system.

Lymph Congestion Relief Oil

2 tablespoons poke root
1 tablespoon fennel seed
½ tablespoon lobelia leaf
¾ cup olive oil
45 drops grapefruit essential oil
15 drops rosemary essential oil

Put the herbs in a glass baking dish and cover with olive oil to a depth of 1 or 2 inches. Bake at 170 degrees F for 4 hours. Allow to cool and then strain. Transfer to bottle of your choice and add the essential oils. Rub 1 teaspoon over the neck glands to help reduce swelling.

Lymphatic-Support Capsules

¾ ounce burdock root
½ ounce figwort leaf
½ ounce violet leaf
¼ ounce stone root

Mix the powdered herbs in a bowl and fill 200 empty capsules. Take 2 capsules twice a day.

Tea for Swollen Glands

1 ounce pipsisssewa leaf
1 ounce cleavers leaf
½ ounce white willow leaf
½ ounce calendula flower
½ ounce hibiscus fruit
½ ounce lemongrass

Mix the herbs in a bowl and store in a glass jar. Make tea by the cup. Steep 1 or 2 teaspoons in 10 ounces of hot water, covered, for 10 minutes. Drink hot, 2 to 3 cups a day for 4 to 5 days.

Care for Babies & Children

I grew up in the antibiotic era and as a child probably took three or four courses of antibiotics each winter. Whenever my throat hurt, my ears ached, or my fever shot up, I would be given the same amoxicillin. Sometimes it was warranted, but many times it was not. As I grew older and began studying herbs and nature-cure traditions, I became more comfortable identifying when I was able to treat myself and when I did indeed need to see my health care practitioner. By the time I had my first child, using herbs seemed only natural to me.

Children respond so much more quickly than adults to medicines of any type. Just a little yarrow and peppermint tea brought my daughter's fevers down, and a little cleavers oil to the throat diminished swollen glands. When I caught a nasty cold when my son was just four weeks old, I drank a tea of boneset, elderflower, echinacea root, and peppermint to fight it and provide my son the protective benefits through my breast milk. I have found that most children relate to plants as healing medicine and often want to know what the herb looks like and how it works. Having this cooperative relationship with patients who want to actively participate in their healing process is quite rewarding.

Many customers come to my herb shop for the first time when they become parents. They are seeking gentle but effective ways to help their children move through day-to-day issues and to relieve discomfort. Herbs can offer a supportive approach to many families' daily health needs. Encourage your children to share the experience with you as you make the recipes in this section. Even when they are babies, you can show them the herbs and how to take them. Our kids are always watching us and gain from positive demonstration.

Guidelines for treating children and babies

- If cold symptoms are present, get on it. Don't delay in treating.

- Always treat a cough aggressively.

- Take a look at what you're wearing before you go outside with your baby or child. If you are wearing a heavy coat and winter hat, your child should be too. Yes, kids run warm, but leaving them exposed to wind and cold is inviting a cold to come in.

- Don't overdress for bedtime.

- Use essential oils in a diffuser to prevent the domino effect when one member of the family gets sick.

- When one member of the family gets sick, be proactive with immune-boosting herbs for everyone else.

Dosage guidelines for children

Any parent who is just learning about herbs needs some guidance to determine the appropriate quantities of herbs for children. The goal is to use a safe quantity of herbs but also use enough to be effective. Use these dosage tables to determine the appropriate quantity of herbs to give a child. And use the dosages given for each of the specific recipes in this section, even if they don't exactly match these general guidelines.

TINCTURE DOSAGES FOR CHILDREN

(if adult dosage is 2 dropperfuls, or 60 drops)

Younger than 3 months*	2 drops
3 to 6 months*	3 drops
6 to 9 months*	4 drops
9 to 12 months*	5 drops
12 to 18 months*	7 drops
18 to 24 months*	8 drops
2 to 3 years*	10 drops
3 to 4 years	12 drops
4 to 6 years	15 drops
6 to 9 years	24 drops
9 to 12 years	30 drops (1 dropperful)

glycerin-only tinctures for 2 years and younger

TEA DOSAGES FOR CHILDREN

(if adult dosage is 1 cup, or 8 ounces)

Younger than 1 year	½ to 3 teaspoons
2 to 4 years	1 to 4 ounces
4 to 7 years	2 to 4 ounces
7 to 11 years	4 to 6 ounces

DOSAGES FOR AGE 12 OR OLDER

PREPARATION	*DOSAGE*
Glycerin tinctures	1 dropperful, 3 or 4 times per day
Syrups	1 teaspoon, 3 to 6 times per day, depending on case

You can also use two equations to determine dosage of any herbal medicine to achieve the percentage of the adult dosage appropriate for a child:

Young's Rule Add 12 to the child's age, and divide the child's age by this total. For example, to determine the dosage for a 4-year-old: 4 + 12 = 16. Then 4 ÷ 16 = 0.25, or one-fourth of the adult dosage.

Cowling's Rule Divide the child's age at his or her next birthday by 24. For example, the dosage for a child who is 3, turning 4 at his next birthday, would be 4 ÷ 24 = 0.16, or about one-sixth of the adult dosage.

Coughs

I'm sure I've said it a hundred times: always always always treat a cough at the first sign of it. This is immensely easier than trying to rid the body of it after it has taken hold. Treat the cough itself with appropriate herbs to alleviate the spasm, irritation, and/or phlegm while simultaneously treating the immune and respiratory systems.

Herbal Cough Syrup

1 ounce coltsfoot leaf

½ ounce mullein leaf

½ ounce pleurisy root

½ ounce wild cherry bark

½ ounce horehound leaf

½ ounce marshmallow root

½ ounce goldenseal root

8 cups water

3 cups cane sugar or honey

¼ cup apple cider vinegar

Put the herbs in a saucepan with the water, bring to a boil, and reduce by half on a medium-low heat. Strain the herbs out and put the brew back into the pan. Add the sugar or honey and gently heat to mix if necessary, stirring continuously. Turn off the heat, add the apple cider vinegar, and allow to cool. Transfer to your container of choice. Give 1 to 2 teaspoons 3 times a day.

Cough-Killer Tea

1 ounce hyssop leaf

1 ounce peppermint leaf

½ ounce coltsfoot leaf

½ ounce mullein leaf

½ ounce marshmallow root

½ ounce licorice root

Mix the herbs in a bowl and store in a glass jar. Make tea by the cup. Steep 1 or 2 teaspoons in 10 ounces of hot water, covered, for 10 minutes. Give 2 or 3 cups a day. If the patient is a baby who is being breastfed, the mother can drink the tea to help support the baby. After 6 months of age you can give 1-teaspoon doses if desired.

Respiratory-Support Tincture

2 teaspoons elecampane root

1 teaspoon goldenseal root

½ teaspoon echinacea root

½ teaspoon rosemary leaf

2 ounces vegetable glycerin

Put the herbs in a 2-ounce jar and add vegetable glycerin to fill. Close tightly and shake well. Keep in a pantry or cupboard for 3 weeks, shaking every day. Strain and transfer to a 2-ounce dropper bottle. Give 1 dropperful 3 times a day at the first sign of a cough or respiratory infection.

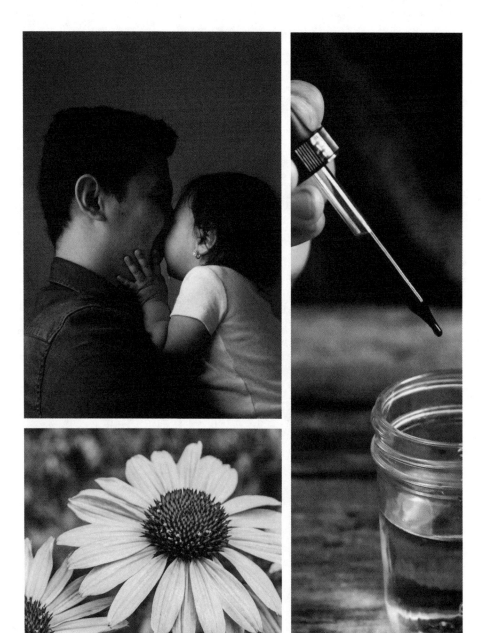

Fever

A true fever in a child can be a very scary experi-ence. Even as a doctor, I have had moments of deep concern when my children have spiked high fevers. When my daughter experienced her first multiple-day fever of 105 degrees F, I questioned myself repeatedly despite my training. I called her pediatrician, who again reminded me that what I was describing was a normal bug. Yes, kids' fevers tend to go high and that is almost always normal, but when you see your child suffering like this it can be a hopeless feeling, and fears can quickly take over. If you decide to reach for the kids' ibuprofen even though you believe in living as naturally as pos-sible, please don't view that as a failure. It isn't going to derail your values should you decide to use mod-ern medicine at certain times as well as the remedies described here.

Fever-Reliever Tea

This tea helps to gently reduce fever and provide comfort to the patient.

1 3/4 ounces yarrow leaf and flower

1 ounce peppermint leaf

1/2 ounce echinacea root

1/2 ounce boneset leaf

1/4 ounce licorice root

Mix the herbs in a bowl and store in a glass jar. Make tea by the cup. Steep 1 or 2 teaspoons in 10 ounces of hot water, covered, for 10 minutes. You may want to start by offering just 6 ounces of the tea. Getting kids to drink tea when they aren't feeling well may take some encouraging, but once they make the connection to how it makes them feel better, it'll get easier.

Cooling Fomentation

40 drops peppermint essential oil

Add the essential oil to cool water in a basin and soak a cotton cloth in it. Wring it out and apply to the forehead.

Fever-Reliever Diffuser Blend

3 milliliters basil essential oil

1 milliliter peppermint essential oil

1 milliliter eucalyptus essential oil

5 milliliter witch hazel extract or fractionated coconut oil

Blend the oils in a 10-milliliter bottle and add 5 drops to your room diffuser.

Head Colds

When your little one can't breathe, no one is sleeping at night. My son recently had a cold with so much phlegm in his little nose that he'd wake up with both nose holes sealed over. Getting the mucus to thin out and drain helps to clear the head, and using essential oils to stimulate the olfactory can move that cold out of the body.

Decongestion Tea

1 ounce peppermint leaf

1 ounce spearmint leaf

1 ounce elderflower

½ ounce echinacea root

½ ounce ginger root

Mix the herbs in a bowl and store in a glass jar. Make tea by the cup. Steep 1 or 2 teaspoons in 10 ounces of hot water, covered, for 10 minutes. Have the child drink while warm.

Cold-Breakup Tincture

2 teaspoons elderberry

1 teaspoon horehound leaf

1 teaspoon boneset leaf

½ teaspoon goldenseal root

½ teaspoon peppermint leaf

2 ounces vegetable glycerin

Put the herbs in a 2-ounce jar and add vegetable glycerin to fill. Close tightly and shake well. Keep in a pantry or cupboard for 3 weeks, shaking every day. Strain and transfer to a 2-ounce dropper bottle. Give 1–2 dropperfuls 4 times a day.

Decongestant Chest Rub

2 tablespoons eucalyptus leaf

1 tablespoon rosemary leaf

1 tablespoon mullein leaf

¾ cup olive oil

½ ounce beeswax

40 drops white thyme essential oil

20 drops pine essential oil

Put the herbs in a glass baking dish and cover with olive oil to a depth of 1 or 2 inches. Bake at 170 degrees F for 4 hours. Allow to cool and then strain. Pour the oil into a saucepan and add the beeswax. Gently heat until the beeswax is melted. Pour into your container of choice and add the essential oils. Rub on the chest as needed.

Sore Throat

A sore throat can make the day hard to get through. When you've ruled out strep throat, these recipes will help to soothe the pain in the gentle way herbs do. But don't forget the good old-fashioned throat gargle using apple cider vinegar or warm water and salt. These traditional ways do the trick!

Throat-Soothe Tea

2 ounces wild cherry bark

1 ounce marshmallow root

½ ounce licorice root

½ ounce thyme leaf

Mix the herbs in a bowl and store in a glass jar. Make tea by the cup. Steep 1 or 2 teaspoons in 10 ounces of hot water, covered, for 10 minutes. Give 3 cups a day until symptoms subside.

Throat-Soothe Spray

2 teaspoons elderberry

2 teaspoons marshmallow root

½ teaspoon echinacea root

½ teaspoon ginger root

1 ounce apple cider vinegar

1 ounce vegetable glycerin

Put the herbs in a 2-ounce jar and add apple cider vinegar and vegetable glycerin to fill. Close tightly and shake well. Keep in a pantry or cupboard for 3 weeks, shaking every day. Strain and transfer to a 2-ounce spray bottle. Spray directly onto the throat multiple times a day.

Throat-Soothe Oil

2 tablespoons chickweed leaf

2 tablespoons sage leaf

1 tablespoon cleavers leaf

¾ cup olive oil

Put the herbs in a glass baking dish and cover with olive oil to a depth of 1 or 2 inches. Bake at 170 degrees F for 4 hours. Allow to cool and then strain. Transfer to your bottle of your choice. Rub 1 teaspoon over external throat/neck area twice daily.

Metric Conversions

FEET	METERS
1	0.3
2	0.6
3	0.9
4	1.2
5	1.5
10	3.0
50	15.2
100	30.5

INCHES	CENTIMETERS
1	2.5
2	5.0
5	12.7

US WEIGHT MEASURE	METRIC EQUIVALENT
1/16 ounce	1.8 grams
1/8 ounce	3.5 grams
1/4 ounce	7.0 grams
1/2 ounce	14.2 grams
3/4 ounce	21.3 grams
1 ounce	28.3 grams
1 1/2 ounces	42.5 grams
2 ounces	56.7 grams
3 ounces	85.0 grams
4 ounces	113.4 grams
8 ounces	226.8 grams
10 ounces	283.5 grams
12 ounces	340.2 grams
16 ounces	453.6 grams

US VOLUME MEASURE	METRIC EQUIVALENT
1/16 teaspoon	0.3 milliliter
1/8 teaspoon	0.5 milliliter
1/4 teaspoon	1.2 milliliters
1/2 teaspoon	2.5 milliliters
1 teaspoon	5.0 milliliters
1 tablespoon (3 teaspoons)	14.8 milliliters
2 tablespoons (1 fluid ounce)	29.6 milliliters
1/8 cup (2 tablespoons)	29.6 milliliters
1/4 cup (4 tablespoons)	59.1 milliliters
1/2 cup (4 fluid ounces)	118.3 milliliters
3/4 cup (6 fluid ounces)	177.4 milliliters
1 cup (16 tablespoons)	236.6 milliliters
1 pint (2 cups)	473.2 milliliters
1 quart (4 cups)	946.4 milliliters

Herbal Suppliers

Dandelion Botanical Company dandelionbotanical.com

Fettle Botanic Supply & Counsel fettlebotanic.com

Foster Farm Botanicals fosterfarmbotanicals.com

Gaia Herbs gaiaherbs.com

Mountain Rose Herbs mountainroseherbs.com

Oregon's Wild Harvest oregonswildharvest.com

Pacific Botanicals pacificbotanicals.com

Radiance Herbs radianceherbs.com

Wise Woman Herbals wisewomanherbals.com

Wonderland Herbs Teas and Spices
wonderlandherbsteasspices.wordpress.com

Botanical Names of Herbs Used

agrimony *Agrimonia eupatoria*

alder buckthorn *Frangula alnus*

alfalfa *Meticago sativa*

angelica *Angelica archangelica*

anise *Pimpinella anisum*

arnica *Arnica montana*

asafoetida *Ferula assa-foetida*

ashwagandha *Withania somnifera*

barberry *Berberis vulgaris*

bilberry *Vaccinium myrtillus*

black cohosh *Actaea racemosa* (also *Cimicifuga racemosa*)

black walnut *Juglans nigra*

blessed thistle *Cnicus benedictus* (also *Centaurea benedicta*)

boneset *Eupatorium perfoliatum*

borage *Borago officinalis*

bupleurum *Bupleurum chinense*

burdock *Arctium lappa*

butcher's broom *Ruscus aculeatus*

calendula *Calendula officinalis*

California poppy *Eschscholzia californica*

caraway *Carum carvi*

cascara sagrada *Frangula purshiana*

catnip *Nepeta cataria*

cat's claw *Uncaria tomentosa*

cayenne *Capsicum annuum*

cedar *Thuja occidentalis*

celandine *Chelidonium majus*

celery *Apium graveolens*

centaury *Centaurium erythraea*

chamomile *Matricaria chamomilla*

chaparral *Larrea divaricata*

chickweed *Stellaria media*

cleavers *Galium aparine*

clove *Syzygium aromaticum*

club moss *Lycopodium clavatum*

coltsfoot *Tussilago farfara*

comfrey *Symphytum officinale*

couch grass *Elymus repens*

cramp bark *Viburnum opulus*

damiana *Turnera diffusa*

dandelion *Taraxacum officinale*

devil's club *Oplopanax horridus*

dong quai *Angelica sinensis*

echinacea *Echinacea purpurea*

elder *Sambucus nigra*

elecampane *Inula helenium*

eleuthero *Eleutherococcus senticosus*

epimedium *Epimedium sagittatum*

eyebright *Euphrasia officinalis*

fennel *Foeniculum vulgare*

fenugreek *Trigonella foenum-graecum*

figwort *Scrophularia nodosa*

fo-ti *Polygonum multiflorum*

frankincense *Boswellia serrata*

gentian *Gentiana lutea*

ginger *Zingiber officinale*

ginkgo *Ginkgo biloba*

goat's rue *Galega officinalis*

goldenseal *Hydrastis canadensis*

gotu kola *Centella asiatica*

grand cactus *Selenicereus grandiflorus*

gravel root *Eupatorium purpureum*

guarana *Paullinia cupana*

hawthorn *Crataegus laevigata*

hibiscus *Hibiscus sabdariffa*

holy basil *Ocimum tenuiflorum*

hops *Humulus lupulus*

horehound *Marrubium vulgare*

horse chestnut *Aesculus hippocastanum*

horseradish *Armoracia rusticana*

horsetail *Equisetum arvense*

hydrangea *Hydrangea arborescens*

hyssop *Hyssopus officinalis*

Jamaican dogwood *Piscidia piscipula*

juniper *Juniperus communis*

kava kava *Piper methysticum*

lady's mantle *Alchemilla vulgaris*

lavender *Lavendula* species

lemon balm *Melissa officinalis*

lemongrass *Cymbopogon* species

licorice *Glycyrrhiza glabra*

linden *Tilia americana*

lion's mane *Hericium erinaceus*

lobelia *Lobelia inflata*

lomatium *Lomatium dissectum*

maca *Lepidium meyenii*

maitake *Grifola frondosa*

marshmallow *Althaea officinalis*

meadowsweet *Filipendula ulmaria*

milk thistle *Silybum marianum*

motherwort *Leonurus cardiaca*

mugwort *Artemisia vulgaris*

mullein *Verbascum thapsus*

myrrh *Commiphora myrrha*

nettle *Urtica dioica*

oatstraw *Avena sativa*

Oregon grape *Mahonia aquifolium*

osha *Ligusticum porteri*

partridge berry *Mitchella repens*

passionflower *Passiflora incarnata*

pau d'arco *Tabebuia avellanedae*

peppermint *Mentha ×piperita*

pine *Pinus pinaster*

pipsissewa *Chimaphila umbellata*

plantain *Plantago major*

pleurisy root *Asclepias tuberosa*

poke *Phytolaca americana*

poplar *Populus tremuloides*

prickly ash *Zanthoxylum clava-herculis*

raspberry *Rubus idaeus*

red clover *Trifolium pratense*

red root *Amaranthus retroflexus*

reishi *Ganoderma applanatum* (also
G. lucidum, *G. oregonense, G. tsugae*)

rhodiola *Rhodiola rosea*

rooibos *Aspalanthus linearis*

rose *Rosa* species

rosemary *Rosmarinus officinalis*

safflower *Carthamus tinctorius*

sage *Salvia officinalis*

saw palmetto *Serenoa repens*

schisandra *Schisandra chinensis*

shatavari *Asparagus racemosus*

shepherd's purse *Capsella bursa-pastoris*

shiitake *Lentinula edodes*

silk tassel *Garrya elliptica*

skullcap *Scutellaria lateriflora*

slippery elm *Ulmus rubra*

spearmint *Mentha spicata*

spilanthes *Spilanthes acmella*

St. John's wort *Hypericum perforatum*

stone root *Collinsonia canadensis*

sumac *Rhus glabra*

thyme *Thymus vulgaris*

tribulus *Tribulus terrestris*

turkey rhubarb *Rheum palmatum*

turmeric *Curcuma longa*

usnea *Usnea barbata*

valerian *Valeriana officinalis*

vervain *Verbena officinalis*

violet *Viola odorata*

vitex *Vitex agnus-castus*

white oak *Quercus alba*

white willow *Salix alba*

wild cherry *Prunus serotina*

wild lettuce *Lactuca virosa*

wild yam *Dioscorea villosa*

wireweed *Sida acuta*

wood bettony *Stachys officinalis*

wormwood *Artemisia absinthium*

yarrow *Achillea millefolium*

yellow dock *Rumex crispus*

yerba santa *Eriodictyon californicum*

yohimbe *Pausinystalia johimbe*

yucca *Yucca glauca*

Further Reading

Buhner, Stephen Harrod. 2012. *Herbal Antibiotics*, 2nd ed. North Adams, MA: Storey.

Crow, Tis Mal. 2001. *Native Plants, Native Healing: Traditional Muskogee Way*. Summertown, TN: Native Voices.

Deitsch, Irene. 2016. *Tussie-Mussies: A Collector's Guide to Victorian Posy Holders*. Palo Alto, CA: Irene Deitsch.

Duke, James A. 2000. *The Green Pharmacy Herbal Handbook*. Emmaus, PA: Rodale.

Gladstar, Rosemary. 2012. *Rosemary Gladstar's Medicinal Herbs: A Beginner's Guide*, 9th ed. North Adams, MA: Storey.

Green, James. 2007. *The Male Herbal: The Definitive Health Care Book for Men and Boys*, 2nd ed. Berkeley, CA: Crossing Press.

Hoffmann, David. 1989. *The Herbal Handbook: A User's Guide to Medical Herbalism*. Rochester, VT: Inner Traditions.

—. 1993. *An Elders' Herbal: Natural Techniques for Health and Vitality*. Rochester, VT: Healing Arts Press.

Kloos, Scott. 2017. *Pacific Northwest Medicinal Plants*. Portland, OR: Timber Press.

Kloss, Jethro. 1939. *Back to Eden*. Loma Linda, CA: Back to Eden Books.

Laufer, Geraldine Adamich. 2000. *Tussie-Mussies: The Language of Flowers*. New York, NY: Workman.

Light, Phyllis D. 2018. *Southern Folk Medicine: Healing Traditions from the Appalachian Fields and Forests*. Berkeley, CA: North Atlantic Books.

Pursell, JJ. 2015. *The Herbal Apothecary: 100 Medicinal Herbs and How to Use Them*. Portland, OR: Timber Press.

—. 2018. *The Woman's Herbal Apothecary: 200 Natural Remedies for Healing, Hormone Balance, Beauty and Longevity, and Creating Calm*. Beverly, MA: Fair Winds Press.

Stuart, Malcolm, ed. 1979. *The Encyclopedia of Herbs and Herbalism*. New York, NY: Grosset and Dunlap.

Acknowledgments

When I get to this point, I always take a moment and reflect back on the process of manifesting the book you hold in your hands. I am flooded with the faces, memories, and environments that were part of its creation. Writing is such an intimate process and each page and where it was written has memories woven throughout.

To all of the support at Timber—Stacee, Sarah, Lorraine, Jacoba, Mike, Vincent, and Hillary—no one could ask for a better team. And of course, Shawn Linehan, my sister friend, you've ruined it for all other photographers because your perfection through the lens is now something I cannot live without. Thank you for your patience, wise counsel, and making my beautiful book. As always, I end with giving thanks to all the teachers, herbalists, plant doctors, and to the plants themselves, for giving me a chance and showing me the way into your world.

Kind regards,

JJ

Photo Credits

Karen Bergstom, 81 bottom
Shawn Linehan, 6, 15, 23, 24, 26, 31, 35, 40, 41, 43, 45, 47, 51, 55, 57, 59, 93
Sarah Milhollin, 82 top
Tom Potterfield, 88 bottom
JJ Pursell, 68a, 78 bottom, 79 bottom

Alamy
bildagentur-online.com/th-foto, 91 bottom

Flickr
Used under a Creative Commons Attribution 0.0 Generic license
Olive Titus, 72 top

Used under a Creative Commons Attribution 2.0 Generic license
Esther Westerveld, page 61 bottom
F. D. Richards, page 62 top
Liz West, 63 top
peganum, 89 bottom
Peter O'Connor, 90 bottom
Quinn Dombrowski, 75 bottom
Wendell Smith, 90 top

iStock
CCeliaPhoto, 75 top
jatrax, 71 bottom
lissart, 66 top
wbritten, 86 bottom
yanmiao, 66 bottom

PublicDomainPictures.net
Suzie Hudon, 67 top
Vera Kratochvil, 64 top

Shutterstock
Carpentry, 74 bottom
jaboo2foto, 80 bottom
JRJfin, 69 bottom
Kseniia Zagrebaeva, 83 top
Kwanjitr, 74 top
Lippert Photography, 78 top
Maxal Tamor, 91 top
Santhosh Varghese, 88 top
Ulada, 63a
Vladimir Melnik, 78 middle

Unsplash
Alejandro Pinero Amerio, 111 bottom left
Allie, 163 bottom left
Amplitude Magazin, 104 top left
Anda Ambrosini, 173 bottom right
Annie Spratt, 20
Arun Sharma, 111 top left
Balu Gaspar, 104 top right
Benjamin Combs, 169 top
Caleb Pudewell, 117 middle right
Chelsea Shapouri, 38, 189 right
Danika Perkinson, 173 bottom left
E S, 155 bottom left
Esther Driehaus, 135 top
Ethan Sykes, 155 top
Farhan Khan, 169 bottom left
Felicia Buitenwerf, 117 bottom left
Gaelle Marcel, 173 top
Geovanny Velasquez, 189 top left
Giulia Bertelli, 121 bottom right
Hemptouch CBD, 121 bottom left
Jazmin Quaynor, 149 bottom left
Jenn Simpson, 135 bottom left
Joe A, 149 top

Jon Tyson, 149 bottom right

Kate Hliznitsova, 121 top left

Kelly Sikkema, 29, 120 top right

Khara Woods, 189 bottom left

Maddi Bazzocco, 104 bottom right

Maude Frederique Lavoie, 163 top, 169 bottom right

Natasha T, 117 bottom right

Oksana Simanovscia, 135 bottom right

Paul Morley, 155 bottom right

Snapbythree My Z, 32

Stacey Gabrielle Koenitz Rozells, 117 top

Stephan H, 67 bottom

Tetiana Bykovets, 111 bottom right

Thomas Park, 111 top right

Tina Witherspoon, 104 bottom left

Wikimedia Commons

Used under the Creative Commons Attribution-Share Alike 1.0 Universal Public Domain Dedication
AnRo0002, 65 bottom, 71 middle, 89 top

Used under the Creative Commons Attribution-Share Alike 2.5 Generic license
Olaf Leillinger, 82 bottom

Used under the Creative Commons Attribution-Share Alike 3.0 German license
MdE, 65 top

Used under the Creative Commons Attribution-Share Alike 3.0 Unported license
Dietrich Krieger, 73 top
Forest & Kim Starr, 87 bottom
H. Zell, 76 top, 79 top

Hajotthu, 76 bottom

James Steakley, 72 bottom

Jean-Pol GRANDMONT, 81 top

Karelj, 69 top

Lazaregagnidze, 84 top

Leoadec, 70 bottom

LuckyStarr, 73 bottom

Qwert1234, 70 top

Ramon F Velasquez, 77 top

Reaperman, 62 bottom

Roland zh, 64 bottom

Schnobby, 77 bottom

Teun Spaans, 71 top

Vladimir Kosolapov, 85 bottom

Used under the Creative Commons Attribution-Share Alike 4.0 International license
Bff, 87 top
R. A. Nonenmacher, 80 top
Salix, 86 top
Vinayaraj, page 61a

Used under the GNU Free Documentation license
Liné1, 84 bottom
Loadmaster (David R. Tribble), 83 bottom

Index

H

hair tonics, 50, 78

hawthorn (*Crataegus laevigata*), 73
about, 73
circulation, 73, 123
heart support, 73
tinctures, 53

hay-fever allergies, 98

Hay-Fever Eyewash, 101

Hay-Fever Tea, 101

headaches, 30, 50, 72, 75, 79, 80, 83, 89, 94, 144, 156

head colds, 144–148, 192–193

Healthy-Circulation Tonic Tea, 123

heart support, 73, 76

hemorrhoids, 64

hemp oil, 134

Herbal Cough Drops, 128

Herbal Cough Syrup, 187

herbal oils, 18, 34–38, 48

Herbal Wound Spray, 131

herb cake, 44

herpes, 75

hibiscus, 153, 179

histamine reactions, 100

holy basil leaf, 141, 147, 151

honey, 50, 51, 109, 126, 128, 129, 152, 161, 172, 187

hops (*Humulus lupulus*)
about, 73
anxiety, 73
digestive complaints, 73
influenza/flu, 157

strobiles, 73

horehound leaf, 128, 129, 145, 161, 187, 193

hormone balance, 16, 69, 76, 90, 91

horny goat weed, 70

horse chestnut, 96, 123

horseradish powder, 167

horseradish root, 152

HPV, 75

hypoxia, 96

hyssop (*Hyssopus officinalis*)
about, 74
bronchitis, 110
chest colds, 116
coughs, 126, 187
fevers, 74
influenza/flu, 74
muscle pain/cramps, 74
respiratory symptoms, 74
sinusitis, 167, 168
sore throat, 172
strep throat, 177

I

ibuprofen, 190

immune boost, 150–154

Immune-Boost Tea, 151

immune defense
capsules, 25–27
care for babies and children, 181–195
dosages for adults, 16–17, 18–19
dosages for children, 183–185

essential oil blends, 28–29

flower essence blends, 32

fomentations, 30–31

herbal oils, 34–37

key ingredients, 59–91

liniments, 38

medicinal teas, 39–43

poultices, 44–45

preparations, 14–17, 20–57

salves, 46–48

sprays, 49

syrups, 50–51

tinctures, 52–55

washes, 56–57

Immune-Defense Balm, 120

Immune-Defense Mushroom Capsules, 119

Immune-System-Up Travel Drops, 154

infection, 72

infertility, 80

inflammation, 49

influenza/flu, 8, 50, 67, 68, 71, 78, 82, 88, 94, 102, 156–159

insomnia, 82, 85, 86

intestinal tract infections, 72

Intestine-Calming Essential Oil Blend, 134

irritable bowel syndrome, 82

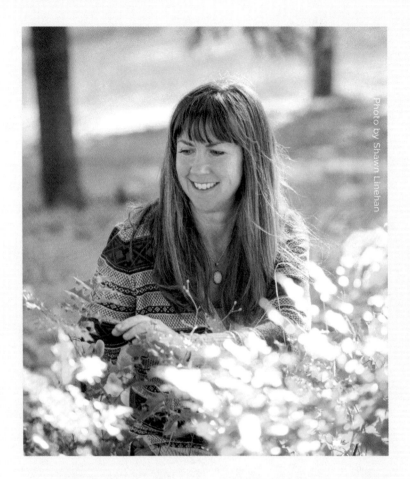

Dr. JJ Pursell is a naturopathic physician and licensed acupuncturist who has worked with medicinal herbs for more than twenty years. She founded The Herb Shoppe and Fettle Botanic Supply & Counsel and currently resides in Oregon, seeing patients, formulating products, supporting fellow entrepreneurs, and spending as much time outside with her family and friends as she can. She's always available for questions at drjjpursell@gmail.com.